The Training Bible:
Proven Programs to Lose Weight Tone, Strengthen And Build Muscle

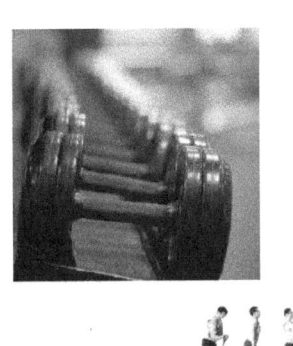
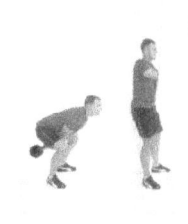

I0426598

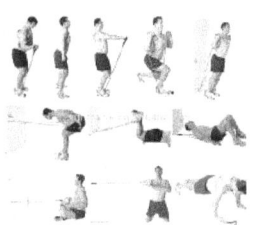

By Master HIT Trainer
David Groscup
IART CFC, IART/Med-Ex High Intensity Trainer
http://www.personal-resistance-trainer.com/
http://drhitshighintensitybodybuilding.blogspot.com/

Table of Contents

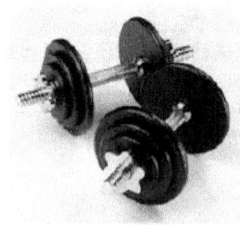

Foreword

My adventures in weight training and the world of weights began when I was 13 years old. I had been involved in martial arts and taken formal training in karate and kung fu. While I thoroughly enjoyed the martial arts, I was bitten by the iron bug the first time I lifted a weight. I was excited to see the new gains in strength and size that resulted from my near daily training.

Unfortunately, like many others, my gains came to a standstill because of excessive training and improper training programs. Around the age of 17 I stumbled across an article written by Mike Mentzer in Muscle Builder Magazine on the subject of HIT, high intensity training. I was doing 12-15 sets of exercises per muscle group, while Mike was using 4-6 sets of all-out effort to train his. For a Mr. Universe competition none-the-less!

Needless to say- I was intrigued! This was completely opposite to everything else I had been reading in all of the muscle magazines. I began training with his programs and began to experience renewed gains in muscle size and strength!

I began to read more articles and amassed additional knowledge on this system of training. I soon realized that healthy eating and a good nutritional supplement program were essential to experience the best gains possible, so I read as much reliable information on the subject of sports supplementation as possible.

I did some powerlifting, and while I enjoyed the lifting of maximum weights in the powerlifts, I was drawn more toward bodybuilding training.

I joined a Nautilus club in the early 80's and experienced a lot of enjoyment from using these machines for training and later on became convinced that machines offered some real advantages for the development of strength, muscle size and fitness.

In more recent years I obtained several trainer certifications, among them IART CFC and IART/Med-Ex HIT Trainer Specialist.

I feel that most types of weight training and fitness training have something to offer the aspiring trainee and have attempted to demonstrate this with my book. I hope you enjoy it thoroughly and apply the principles in your training for the best results.

Introduction

It becomes very difficult to weed through the countless articles in muscle magazines, blogs and websites and come up with effective routines to develop your physique, whether it is for health reasons, a bodybuilding contest or to achieve a lifetime goal of getting in shape and building muscle.

The problem with the muscle mags is the routines espoused by the champions in them are geared for bodybuilders using anabolic steroids or other dangerous growth hormones. Natural bodybuilders aren't going to experience nearly the same results so many of them are going to become discouraged and quit training, which is a shame because the best method for getting and staying in shape is weight training. And it of course is the best and only method for maximizing muscle growth, as you will see in this manual.

What is the ideal amount of reps and sets to experience sustainable muscular growth?

While there is a specific outline of scientifically derived answers to this question, one must also take into consideration how long a trainee has been working out, what his/her recuperative capabilities are as well as other factors.

There will be some trial and error before an ideal combination of amount of sets, reps and days of rest are determined. A great method to use is to train with the routines in this manual and fine-tune them to fit your recuperative abilities. After training a particular body part rest for seven days before training the muscle group again. If you are still sore try adding an additional day or two prior to repeating training. In most cases, seven days should be sufficient.

How important is muscular contraction during training?

As you stroll through gyms and observe trainees of all types and persuasions, you will encounter many different methods of training. You will also observe terrible exercise form used in the exercises, such as barbells swinging with arched backs in the barbell curl, bars being bounced off the chest during bench presses and rapid downward movement in the barbell squat. Most of this is the result of attempts to stroke their ego(s) by using heavier weights than the next guy or gal in their exercises.

The problem with this is the extreme force it places on your joints and tendons, which can lead to career-ending injuries, including muscle tears,

ripped tendons and the like. Not very conducive to a healthy training career is it?

This lack of proper exercise performance also leads to a lesser-than-ideal stimulation of the muscle, which undermines the main focus of bodybuilding training, which is to build bigger, stronger muscles.

In this book we will take a look at the best way to maximize the benefits of your training by increasing the intensity of your working muscle's contractions, thereby utilizing the most fibers you can during an exercise.

The benefits of maximizing muscular contractions in your training

Using proper exercise performance to increase muscular contraction in your exercises activates more muscle fibers than normally possible, leading to far more muscle exhaustion. More muscle exhaustion equals a greater response from your body to rebuild your muscles from the micro damage that occurred during exercise.

Remember, the main concern with bodybuilding training is not how much weight you can lift but how a weight is lifted. After you have been training for a while you will be able to focus the resistance on the muscle and make the weight seem much heavier than it actually is. This is a skill that most trainees lack but is essential if you want to make it to the advanced ranks of bodybuilding.

To practice this, lift a weight, and while slowly raising it, relax all of the muscles not involved in the exercise and concentrate all of the resistance on the muscle being trained. Lower the weight in much the same fashion. With time you will become skilled at this and experience new results while not straining yourself continuously to lift heavier weights.

Ways to increase muscular contraction

Exercise Performance

The way you perform exercises makes a big difference in the results that you experience from your training. When training, make sure to perform exercises in a slow, deliberate fashion to keep pressure on the muscles. I list some examples below:

Dumbbell concentration curl

Curl the dumbbell up toward your shoulder. Instead of using a rapid motion, curl the weight to a count of four. At the top of the movement do six short

"burn reps" and hold the weight at the top for five seconds before returning it to the beginning position. Repeat for the desired amount of reps.

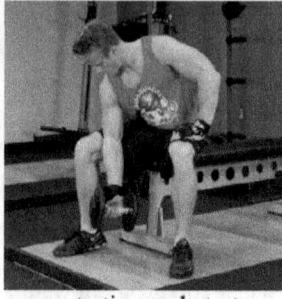 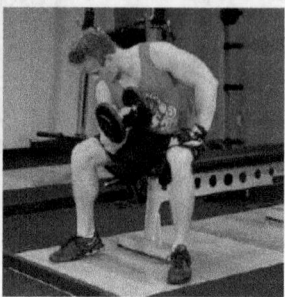

concentration curl-start   finish

By performing concentration curls in this fashion you increase the contraction force in your biceps muscles by activating more muscle fibers.

When you begin an exercise your body uses an initial muscle fiber bank to begin lifting the weight. As you progress, those muscle fibers tire and new ones take over the effort. This effect is magnified by the use of slow speed during exercise. The burn reps at the top of the rep cause a cramping effect, leading to additional fiber stimulus. And finally, the static hold exhausts nearly all of the muscle's remaining fibers.

An exercise combination that is effective at activating maximum muscle fibers for biceps training is:

- **Standing barbell curl**-1 set of 8 individual static holds done in the following fashion. Pick a weight that allows you to hold the barbell at the point of maximum contraction (the point ¾ of the way up) and hold the weight motionless for 20 seconds. This should be done with a weight that begins to descend at the 20-second mark. Return the weight to the start position and after resting for ten seconds, repeat for a total of 8, 20 second holds with a 10 second rest in between. After the initial 2-3 holds it will be necessary to reduce the weight so you are able to complete a full 20-second hold.

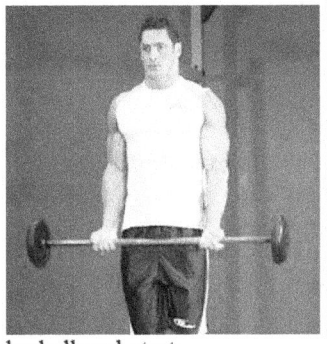 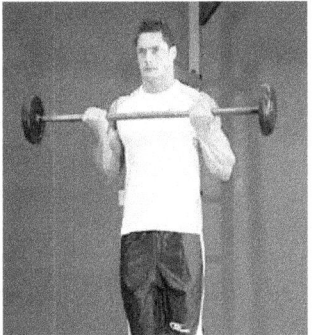

barbell curl-start   finish

- **Partial cable pulldowns-**1 set of 12 reps. Using a palms-facing grip pull the bar to your midsection. Let the bar back one third of the way and do two reps in that zone. Beginning at the middle position, do three reps before completing a final three reps in the top third zone. Use weights that cause you to go to complete muscular exhaustion.

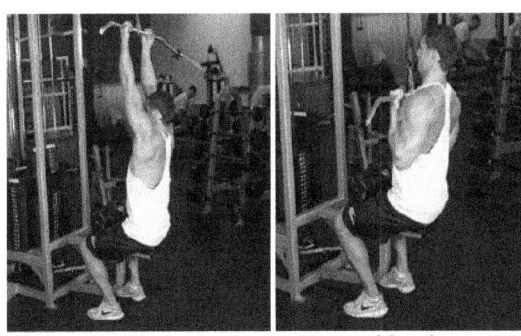

cable pulldowns-start   mid-point

- **Behind-head cable curls-**1 set of 10 reps. While sitting on a bench grab a two-handed rope attachment using a hammer curl grip and curl the rope along the side of your head to the back. Go to failure using a random series of "burn" reps at several different areas of the movement.

Use the following effective routine for the shoulder muscle group:

- **Bent-over dumbbell laterals-** 1 set of 12 reps. Grab a dumbbell in each hand and lean over until you are parallel with the floor. Keeping your arms slightly bent, raise them until they are even with your shoulders. Return to the start position and repeat for the desired rep count. The temptation is to use momentum with this movement, but don't! Go to muscular exhaustion before moving to the next exercise.

- **Front cable raises-** 1 set of 12 reps. Grab a stirrup handle after selecting a weight that causes exhaustion at 12 reps and raise the handle up to a point six inches higher than the top of your head. Your arms should be slightly bent and out in front of you throughout the exercise.

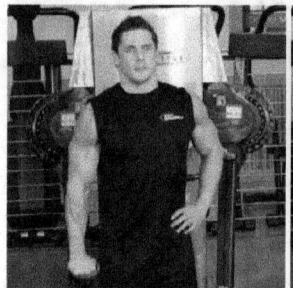 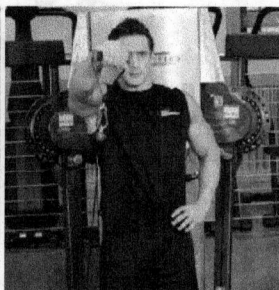

front cable raise-start   finish

- **Seated machine presses-** 1 set of eight static holds with a 10 second rest between reps. Select a weight that allows you to barely hold the press arm for 20 seconds at the point just prior to lockout. Hold the machine press arm in this position for 20 seconds before returning it to the start position. You will need to reduce the weight with each succeeding rep or you will be unable to complete the 20-second hold.

These variables can be used with all body parts to increase training results. Some variations will need to be made at times due to body mechanics but through experience that will become second nature.

HIT- Frequency and Volume

One often-misunderstood ingredient in a bodybuilder's training program is the correct dosage of exercise needed for optimal muscle growth. In other words: the question of how often to train, as well as the number of sets and reps. The temptation is to follow the belief that more is better (i.e. if "x" amount of sets and reps are working, then more will work better-right?). The goal should be to find the optimum amount of training needed to elicit the best results in both muscle growth and conditioning.

There are two points to consider. The first is the frequency of training for an individual muscle group. The second point is the overall rate (volume) of training and the effect that it has on the central nervous system (CNS).

If your program is based on the high volume approach and you are a natural bodybuilder, a small muscle group such as the arms, should be trained hard once per week with a more moderate session spaced several days apart. This is due to the fact that your arms are involved in training every upper body

part and receive a lot of work as a result. Larger muscle groups, such as the chest, legs and back can handle a much more rigorous workload due to their size. Therefore, they can be trained relatively hard twice per week with the high volume approach.

When using a high intensity protocol (HIT), which is the type of training I specialize in, we must shift gears substantially. This method trains muscles with maximum intensity most of the time. About the only time it doesn't is during Intensity Cycling—a period when sub-failure training is used to confuse the body in order to make maximum intensity efforts more effective.

There are several stages of training: beginning, intermediate and advanced.

During the beginning stage small muscle groups such as arms are trained with 3-4 total sets. The large muscle groups (chest, legs and back) are trained using 4-5 total sets with sub-failure training. At this stage, it is more important to learn proper form in all of the exercises rather than worry about making gains.

As soon as the exercises are mastered one advances to the intermediate stage where the set count is reduced to 2-3 sets for small groups and 3-4 sets for large groups. The number of sets used depends on the ability of the trainee to generate maximum intensity. It is best to train harder with less sets. All sets are taken to the point of momentary muscular failure; that is until no more full reps can be completed. In all exercises use good smooth form with no momentum.

After training for 4-6 months you progress to the advanced program. Small muscle groups are trained with 1-2 sets, while large muscle groups are trained using 2-3 sets total. All sets should be taken to the point of momentary muscular failure. After that a high intensity variable, such as forced reps, should be used every other set in order to push the effort past failure.

Now that we have established the outline for progression in HIT, we will focus on the proper frequency of training. Since HIT greatly taxes the muscles and central nervous system it is often necessary to reduce the number of sessions that each muscle group is trained.

A trainee's recuperation level must be taken into consideration as well. Each person's body has it's own capacity for work. A lot of it depends on conditioning and the intensity of effort put forth during training. Some trial and error will have to take place, but overall the guidelines are to train each body part once every seven to ten days. After resting your muscles for seven days attempt another session.

If you are dragging a bit or your weights used during your exercises have dropped try adding an extra 2-3 days between workouts. Since you will be training each group once every 7-10 days your body should be able to recuperate fully.

Depending on your training split, the entire body should be trained in 2-3 sessions over the 7-10 days. This is enough to keep your conditioning high and your muscles growing both larger and stronger.

Let's look at some sample training programs.

This first one is a great leg program:

- Leg extensions, 1 set of 15-20 reps to failure
- Leg presses, 1 set of 12 reps to failure
- Negative-only leg press:

Load the weight approximately 40% heavier than you normally use in this exercise. Using the assistance of a partner or your own arms, press the plate to the point of full extension. Use your left leg only to lower the plate down to the start position. Repeat with your right leg and so on until you can no longer control the downward motion of the machine safely.

Here is a great arm routine:

- Incline dumbbell curls,1 set of 8-10 reps to failure
- Negative-only standing dumbbell curls.

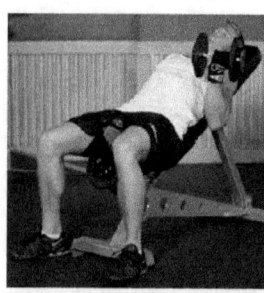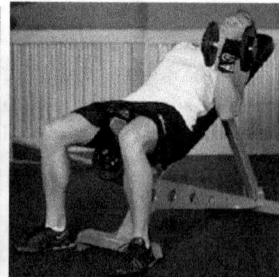

incline dumbbell curl-start   finish

Complete one set of 8 negative reps until unable to control the downward movement. Use a set of 'bells heavy enough to allow a maximum of 8 negatives. Have a partner lift the weights for you or cheat them up; then lower to a count of 8 and repeat.

- Triceps cable pressdowns:1 set of 8-10 reps to failure

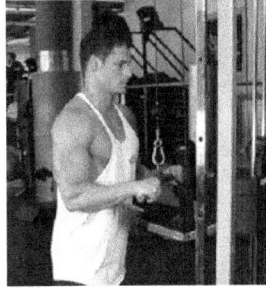 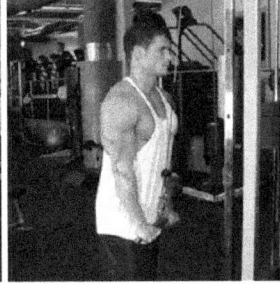

triceps pressdowns-start   finish

Make sure to keep your elbows against your sides throughout the exercise in order to keep the tension on your Triceps.

- Close-grip bench presses: 1 set of 10 reps to failure

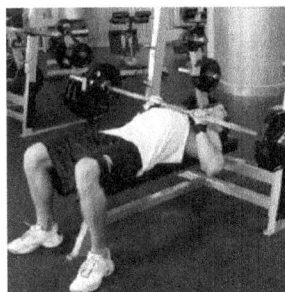 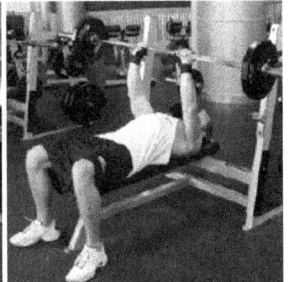

close-grip bench press-start   finish

After completing 10 reps have your partner give you just enough assistance to enable you to complete an additional 3-4 reps. These are forced reps which provide you with the capability of taking your set past the point of normal failure, which is a great way to hammer your triceps to new growth!

- Seated barbell or dumbbell wrist curls, 1 set of 12-15 reps to failure followed by:
- 1 set of reverse wrist curls, 12-15 reps.

You should get a real burn in your forearms after completing these two sets.

These two training routines are a great example of productive HIT programs—good examples of a typical outline for a large and small muscle group.

The other large muscle groups, the chest and back, should follow similar routines to those performed for the legs; simply insert the appropriate exercises for each. Abdominals and lower back (the core), traps and neck are examples of small muscle groups.

Planned training layoffs

After you have been training for a number of months, it is a great idea to take a break so as to allow your body full recuperation from the intense training. Many bodybuilders will tell you that you will lose strength and size, but in most cases you won't.

In fact, most if not everyone will gain some size and strength after a 1-2 week layoff. This is because many people are over-training and need to rest their muscles so they have a chance to grow and recuperate.

Another by-product is your body will no longer be hardened to the intense training. It will begin to respond very positively once you resume working out.

The human system is very efficient at adapting to the stresses placed upon it and quickly adapts to training at maximum intensity. By resting for a short time from your workouts you disrupt the status quo and your body quickly adjusts to your respite from training.

The time off also allows your muscles to completely rebuild and reload with glycogen, creatine and other energy boosters. After the layoff when you resume hard training your body will no longer be accustomed to high intensity effort and you will begin to make gains again, such as you experienced when you first began training.

Alteration of volume and intensity

As mentioned before, your body quickly becomes accustomed to high intensity training—usually after 4-6 months of steady effort. When this happens gains in muscle size and strength will likely cease or at least slow considerably.

To restart gains we must lower the intensity by taking our sets to the point of sub-failure; in other words, end our sets one rep prior to momentary muscular failure. We will also need to slightly increase our set count to reflect the lower concentration of effort.

An arm workout is as follows:

Dumbell Curls-1 set of 8 reps

Supersetted with
Dumbell Concentration Curls-1 set of 12 reps
Do two complete supersets

Lying Barbell Triceps Extensions-1 set of 10 reps
Supersetted with
Cable Triceps Kickbacks-1 set of 8 reps
Do two complete supersets

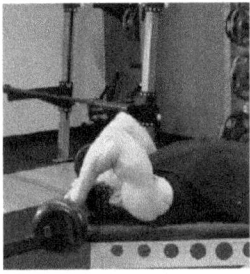 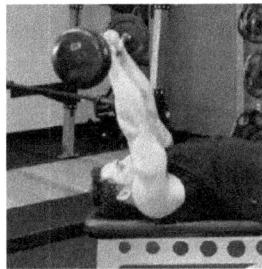

lying barbell triceps extensions-start   finish

Do both supersets with no rest between exercises and carry them to one rep shy of muscular failure.

Continue training your arms with this program for 3-4 weeks then cycle them back to maximum intensity by carrying the sets to failure.

HIT Variables

The routines in this manual contain many different techniques used to increase the intensity of effort. These are called HIT variables and are explained at length in my book, DR. HIT's Effective High Intensity Variables, which is available at Amazon at the following web address: www.amazon.com/author/davidgroscup. I have books on chest and arm training available there as well.

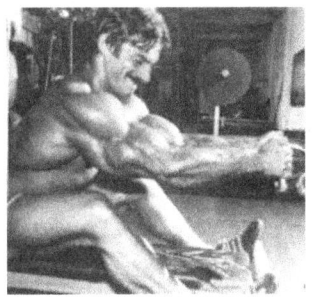

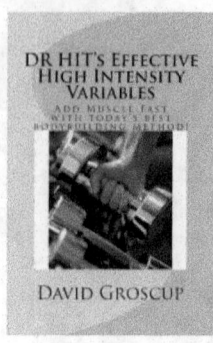

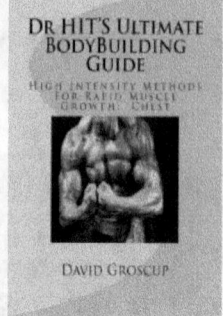

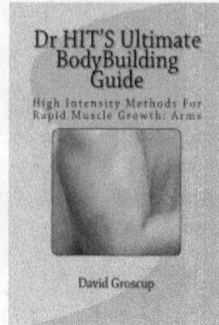

Since HIT variables are explained in detail in my other books, I will not be repeating description of the variables here.

These routines are based on the HIT protocol, which has been shown in scientific studies to be the most efficient method to build muscle fast. I will list single joint and multi-joint exercises for each muscle group near the end of the book. Feel free to substitute alternative exercises from those lists as desired. Use only exercises from the same classification because that is integral to the program's success.

Prior to each workout warm up thoroughly by using a multi-joint exercise. Use a light-moderate resistance and complete 15 reps. Don't actually train the muscle as that compromises its ability to perform during work sets. It's a good idea to repeat a second set using a slightly heavier poundage to make sure you are completely warmed up and condition your muscles to lifting a heavier weight.

Selection of Weight Resistance in Training

Proper selection of weight to use in an exercise is very important to avoid injury and provide the trainee with the results desired.

As a general rule the rep range for strength training is 3-5 reps, the range for hypertrophy or muscle growth increase and strength increase is 6-10 reps.

The following table gives you a good guideline to determine the weight you need to use for the required reps in an exercise. Of course you always attempt to exceed that as a strength increase often occurs prior to an increase in the size of a muscle.

To use this table you will need to determine your one rep max in each exercise. Please warm up thoroughly before attempting this and be careful.

Do not try to go for an all out effort as we are looking for a good starting point only.

The percentage of load in the left column is the percentage of your maximum weight that you can complete for one rep. The column on the right indicates the number of repetitions that normally can be completed with that percentage of one rep maximum.

So for instance, if our goal were to perform eight reps in an exercise, we would use 80% of our one rep maximum.

% Load	Repetitions
60	17
65	14
70	12
75	10
80	8
85	6
90	5
95	3
100	1

On every set try to increase the amount of reps and weight you are using. This is called The Double Overload Principle. The best way to increase the resistance is to add weight to the barbell, dumbbell or machine in small increments. Often, this may be 1.25 or 1.5 lbs.

Aim to increase the amount of reps in the set every time as you increase the weight. While this may seem like a trivial amount of weight, think how much you could increase the amount of weight you are using over the period of a year.

Another way of overloading your muscles is to increase the tension time or repetitions of a set with a given weight. Say you can complete 8 reps in a set of barbell curls with 80 lbs. The next time you train with the barbell curl you should try and increase the rep count of the set to 9 or 10. Of course be sure to use the same good form during the set. The last thing you want to do is sacrifice good form just to use more weight.

After increasing the rep count to 10 add weight to the bar, which should cause you to have to decrease your rep count to 8. During the next training session you should try to increase the rep count to 9 or 10 again. Keep repeating this procedure and remember, as you increase your strength, you will be increasing your muscle size. You will be able to add more weight with this method than the previous one as you will be decreasing the reps when you add the weight initially, then working on increasing the rep count the next workout.

The reason we increase the weight in such small increases is because of the Golgi Tendon Reflex. This is a defense mechanism your body uses to protect itself against injury. If you increase the weight drastically you will be unable to properly contract your muscles to lift the weight. This prevents muscle and tendon tears. If you increase the weight in small increments, the weight will feel no different than it did the workout prior, allowing you to consistently make gains.

Micro Loading Resistance For More Effective Strength Increases

One of the best ways to add weight to either a barbell, dumbbell or weight machine is through Micro Loading. Instead of adding larger increases of weight to the resistance used in an exercise, which often leads to failure to increase the weight, you can add weight in small, almost undetectable increases.

Typically, the smallest weight plate available to use is the 1.25 lb. plate, which means that 2.5 lbs. is being added to the amount lifted. While this is certainly not a large amount of weight, it sometimes can be too much of an increase at one time.

There are newer plates, which are called Micro Plates that come in ½ and 5/8 lbs. each. This allows you to add just one plate to a machine stack, which will give you an increase as small as ½ lb. or use one plate on both sides of a barbell or dumbbell, which increases the weight by only 1 lb.

This allows you to implement regular increases in resistance each training session. If you look at what this means on an annual basis, you can see that over a year you will see large increases in strength even though you are only increasing the weight by 1 lb. per week. That's 52 lbs. per year!

Obviously, you will reach sticking points like you did before but I have found this to be a very effective method. There are various companies that manufacture these plates; therefore they should be obtainable through your local weight training supply store or online. You can also make them yourself with one inch holed washers from Home Depot or Lowes.

Determine what weight you want to make and weigh the washers to determine how many to buy for the weight desired. Braze weld them together to make one heavier washer. Make two of each weight so you have a set to use on your barbells and dumbbells. The ones pictured here are a set I made from three, one inch holed washers that I braze-welded together. They each weigh 5/8 lb., so I am able to increase the weight on my bar by 1.25 lb. at a time.

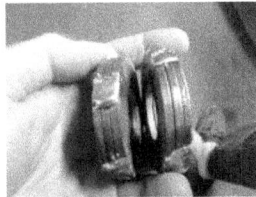

A good rule of thumb is to attempt to add ½-1 lb. per week to exercises for smaller body parts like the arm muscles.

For example: Week one, Barbell Curl 60 lbs. for eight reps.
Week two, 61.25 lbs. for eight reps.
Week three, 62.5 lbs. for eight reps after removing the micro plates and adding two, 1.25 lb. plates.
Week four, 63.75 after adding the micro plates to the bar while keeping the 1.25 lb. plates on.

Keep using this format until you reach your goals for the weight on a given exercise. This system works well for selectorized stack machines as well.

HIT Training Routines

Legs

Reverse pre-exhaustion routine
Front barbell squats-1 set 12-15 reps to failure
No rest
Leg presses-1 set 15 reps to failure
No rest
Leg extensions-15 reps to failure

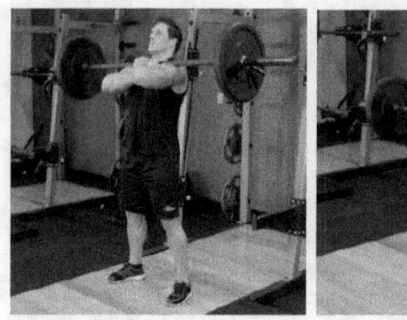 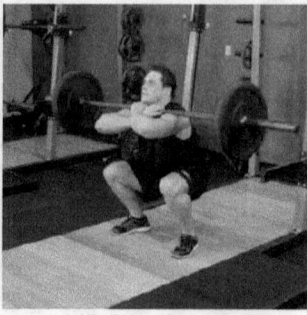

front barbell squats-start   finish

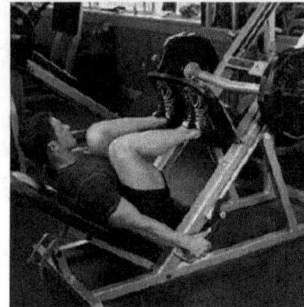 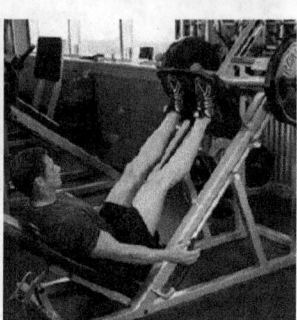

leg press-start   finish

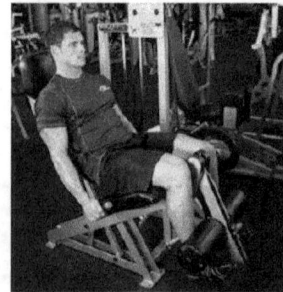 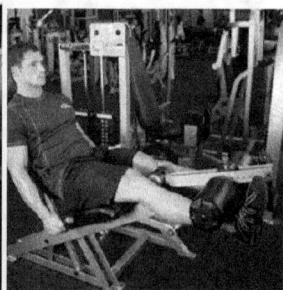

leg extensions-start   finish

This routine begins with two multi-joint exercises, which train the entire leg and hip region. The squats utilize the back muscles to assist the legs in completing the squats. The leg presses train the legs with the hips assisting. The final exercise, leg extensions, isolates the thigh muscles completing them to muscular exhaustion.

Traditional pre-exhaustion routine
Leg extensions-1 set 12-15 reps to failure-several "burn" reps at end of set
No rest
Barbell squats-1 set 12 reps to failure
No rest
Dumbbell lunges-1 set 12 reps each leg

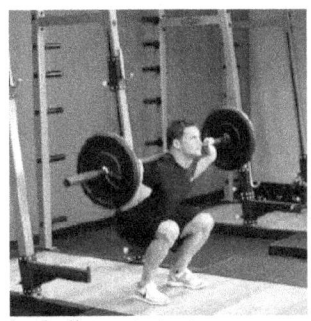 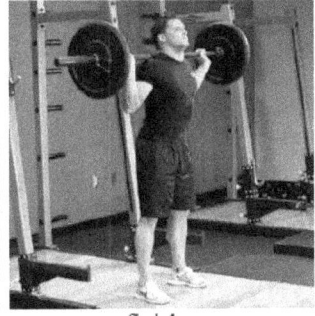

barbell squat-start   finish

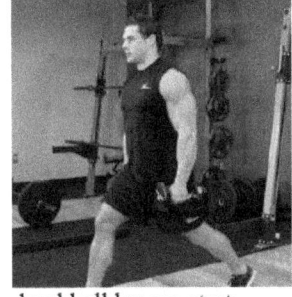 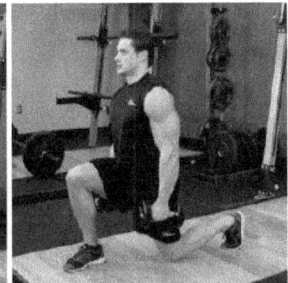

dumbbell lunges-start   finish

Negative-only routine
Leg press-negative only-1 set 12 negative reps to failure
Select a weight that is 40% heavier than you use during traditional leg press sets. Have a training partner assist you in pressing the footplate to the point just prior to lockout. Lower the weight all the way until your knees are completely drawn in to your chest using a count of eight. Pause for one second and then repeat for a total of 8 reps.
No rest
Leg extensions-negative only-1 set 15 reps.
Set the weight at an amount 40% heavier than you normally use in this exercise. Have your partner lift the extension arm to the point of full extension. Being very careful, take all of the pressure onto your legs and lower to a count of 8. Repeat for a total of 15 reps.

Power routine
Squats
Set 1-8 reps @70% 1rm
Set 2-6 reps @80% 1rm
Set 3-4 reps @90% 1rm
Set 4-2 reps @95% 1rm
Set 5-1 rep @100% 1rm

Rest 2-3 minutes between sets depending on your conditioning and experience level.

Go down to the point of your legs being parallel with the floor-no lower as that could cause injury.

Leg presses
Set 1-6 reps @80% of 1rm
Set 2-4 reps @90% of 1rm
Set 3-2 reps @95% of 1rm

Rest 2-3 minutes between sets as noted above. You may go to the point of lockout on these but don't remain in that position for more than one second.

Partials Reps routine
Partial rep squats-1 set 15 partial reps
Using a power rack set the pins so you can lower no more than one third of the way. Load the barbell with a weight much heavier than normal-one that allows you to complete 5 reps to exhaustion. Rack the weight and reset the pins to the mid-point position. Do 5 reps from mid-point to ¾ of the way up. Rest 3 minutes then lift the bar off the pins after setting them at the bottom position. Do a total of 5 reps to finish the set.

Rest 2 minutes then repeat. Do a total of three of these sets per session.

Partial rep leg extensions-1 set of 15 reps
Do 5 reps in the bottom $1/3^{rd}$ of the exercise. Continue the set by doing 5 reps in the middle $1/3^{rd}$ and finishing by performing 5 reps in the top, or final $1/3^{rd}$ of the exercise. Squeeze at the top of each rep for one second to increase muscle fiber tension.

Hamstring Routine
Leg curls- 1 set of 15 reps to failure
Perform these on a lying, standing or seated machine
No rest
Standing barbell stiff-legged deadlift- 1 set 12 reps to failure
Lock your knees, bend over and grab the barbell. Use either a cross grip or a over handed grip on the bar. Stand up straight with the bar keeping your arms fully extended. Repeat for the required rep count.

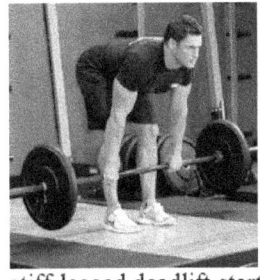 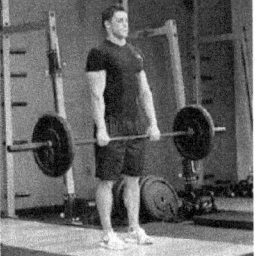

stiff-legged deadlift-start   finish

Calf routine
Standing calf raises-1 set of 15 reps to failure
Use a selectorized standing calf machine if available. If not, a set of dumbbells-one in each hand- is fine. Or if you prefer, hold a dumbell in your left hand as you train the left calf. Switch hands and train your right calf muscle. Make sure to lower all the way down for a good stretch and extend your foot all the way up to train the muscle through the full range of motion.
Seated calf raises-1 set of 15 reps to failure
This exercise trains the soleus muscle, the large muscle behind the calf, or gastrocnemius muscle. This muscle adds size to your calf and gives it a nice full appearance.

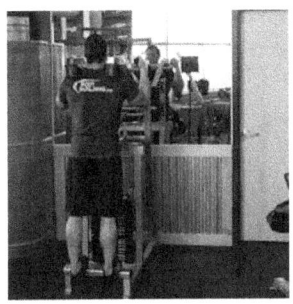 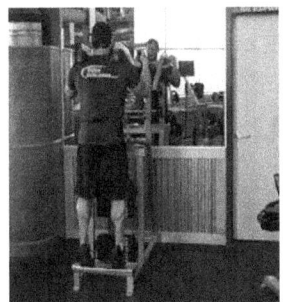

standing calf raises-start   finish

Despite being one of the smaller muscle groups, the calf demonstrates enormous strength potential. Many people can lift the entire weight stack on a calf machine or support several people during a donkey calf raise.

This is due to the tendon insertion points on both ends of the calf, giving it a great leverage advantage. This coupled with a short range of motion, give the calf muscle its unique strength.

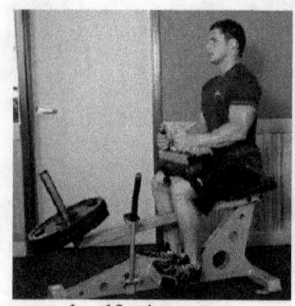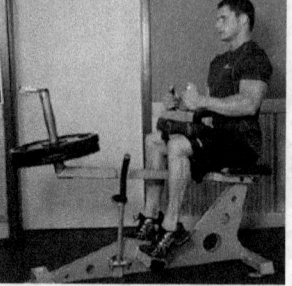

seated calf raises-start   finish

Calf routine #2

Leg press machine toe presses- 1 set of 12 reps to failure

Lock your knees and place the front of your foot on the bottom of the press plate. Get a good stretch by letting the weight push your feet toward you and press your toes as far forward as you can. Repeat for a total of 12 reps.

Donkey calf raises-1 set of 15 reps to failure

Use one or more partners on your back to add weight to the movement. Place your hands on a bench as you lean over perpendicular to the floor. Lock your knees and get a complete stretch as you lower your heels toward the floor. Extend your heels up as far as you can to get a full contraction. Repeat. There is a donkey calf machine with a selectorized weight stack, which is perfect for this exercise.

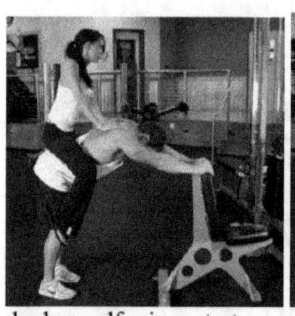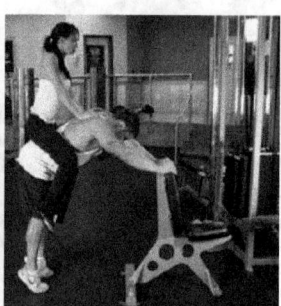

donkey calf raises-start   finish

Abdominals and related muscle groups

Your abs and the muscle groups that constitute your "core" are very important for posture, injury prevention and balanced physique development. In virtually every exercise movement, as well as in daily life, your "central muscles" form a base for your other muscles to work and project power. In addition to the abdominals, the obliques, intercostals and other muscles are included in this group.

The old school method, and the one still most accepted, way of training this group is with a high rep, high set program. This is thought to burn off fat better than a lower rep, lower set routine.

Companies manufacturing products that guarantee to isolate your ab muscles have promoted the theory of spot reduction of fat extensively and spot reduce fat off your abdominal area. The truth is that in order to lose fat you need to burn more calories than you consume.

Make sure to follow a rational approach when developing eating habits. Eat plenty of lean protein with a blend of complex carbohydrates such as fruits and vegetables and a fair amount of good fats such as olive or fish oil. It is ok to deviate from your healthy diet at times and have some ice cream or some other "bad snack." The best long-term approach is to avoid "going on a diet" as that eventually leads to overeating and weight gain.

Abdominals

Ab Routine #1
Ab crunches- 1 set of 15 reps to failure
Lying knee raises- 1 set of 15 reps to failure
Side bends with dumbbells- 1 set of 20 reps
Grab a dumbbell in each hand and hold it at arm's length. Stand straight and bend down to the left while keeping your legs straight. Straighten up and bend down to your right side. Repeat by alternating each side for a total of 20 reps each side.

This is a tri-set routine so there is no rest between exercises. As soon as you complete one exercise go immediately to the next one.

Note: Isolate the abdominals by relaxing all of the muscles not involved in the crunch and knee raise movements. Focus on tensing your upper ab musculature during the crunches and your lower ab muscles during the leg raise movement.

As you become stronger ad weight via ankle weights in the knee raises and by holding a weight plate behind your head or on your chest during the crunches. It is recommended that you add only enough weight to cause you to achieve muscular exhaustion at 15 reps to avoid thickening your ab muscles too much as that can lead to a larger midsection instead of the much sought after tapered waste.

Ab Routine #2
Hanging leg raises- 1 set of 15 reps
No rest
Incline bench sit-ups- 1 set of 15 reps
Rest for one minute then repeat the cycle. Do not swing during the hanging leg raises as momentum takes the stress off the ab muscles, which is the opposite of what we are attempting to achieve.
Side bends with bar- 1 set of 2 minutes
Grab an unloaded barbell and place it on your shoulders behind your neck. Begin standing straight. Twist to the left then right for one complete rep. Continue for a total of 2 minutes.

Ab Routine #3
Machine crunches- 1 set of 12 reps to failure
Sit in the ab crunch machine and place your chest against the front pad. Begin by curling the movement arm down to the finish position using your ab muscles alone. A good way to do this is to relax all of your other muscles while performing the exercise.
No rest
Hanging knee raises- 1 set of 15 reps to failure
Using both hands hang from a chin-up bar. Bring both knees up to your chest and hold for one second before lowering to the start position. Make sure to use no momentum during the exercise.
Exercise wheel floor rolls- 1 set of 12 reps
Kneel on the floor and hold an ab wheel on the floor in front of you. Keep your arms straight and roll the wheel out in front of you on the floor. Extend your upper body out in front of you. Using your ab muscles pull yourself back to the start position. Repeat for a total of 12 reps.

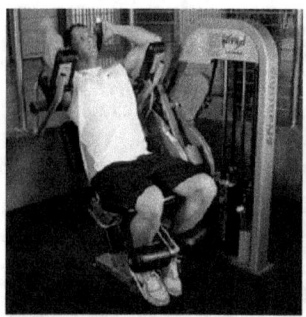
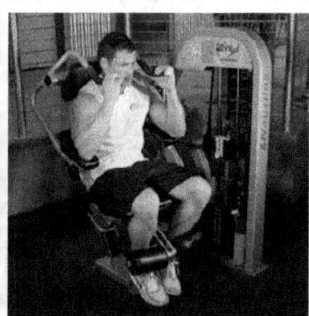

ab crunches-start   finish

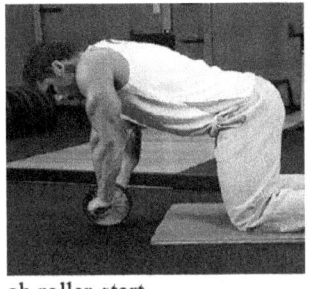 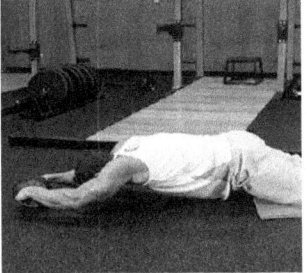

ab roller-start   mid-point

Chest

Chest Routine #1
Machine Flyes- 1 set of 12 reps to failure
Sit in a pek dek or flye machine and grab the handles. Using an arc motion bring the handles directly in front of you, stopping the handles just prior to them touching. Pause for one second then return to the start position. Repeat for a total of 12 reps.
No rest
Decline Bench Press- 1 set of 10 reps to failure
Lie on a decline bench with a barbell loaded with a weight that causes muscular exhaustion at 12 reps. Lift the barbell off the rack and lower it to your chest at a point an inch or so above your nipples. Pause for one second then press it to the point just prior to the lockout position. Repeat for a total of 12 reps.
Bar dips- 1 set of 10 reps to failure
Lean forward and lower to a full stretch then press yourself upward to the point just prior to lockout. Repeat for a total of 10 reps. It is important to lean forward during this exercise. If you use an erect position you will place the majority of the emphasis on your triceps muscles instead of your chest.

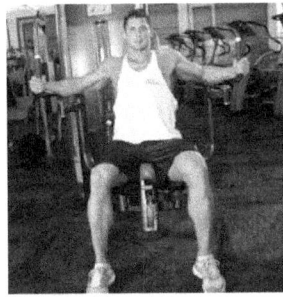 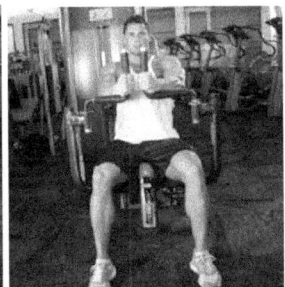

pec fly-start   finish

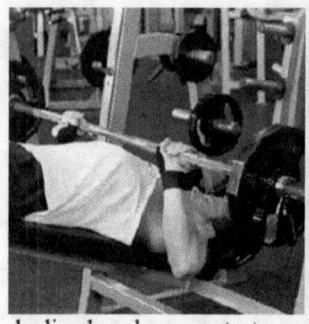 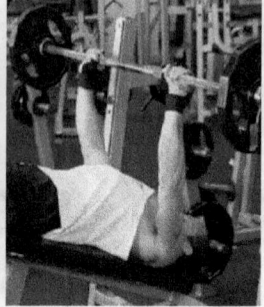

decline bench press-start   finish

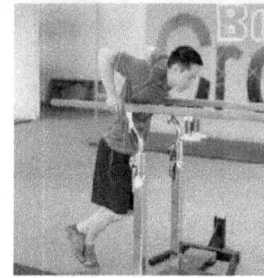 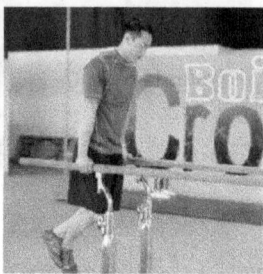

bar dips-start   finish

Chest Routine #2

Incline bench flyes- 1 set of 10 reps to failure

Lower two dumbbells to get a full stretch in your chest. Pause one second, then using an arcing motion, bring them to the point just prior to them touching. Pause one second then repeat.

Incline machine bench press- 1 set of 8 reps plus 3 forced reps

Lie on an incline bench, grab a barbell and press it to the point just prior to lockout. After failing at 8 reps have your training partner provide you with just enough assistance to complete an additional 3 reps. It is important for your partner to only give enough assistance to allow completion of the reps and use a smooth transition between assistance and non-assistance during the rep. The forced rep assistance is only given during the positive portion of the rep.

Negative-only bar dips- 1 set of 8 reps

Use a weight belt to add weight if necessary as you will need to use a resistance that is 40% heavier than you use during a normal set of dips. Beginning at the top of the movement lower yourself to a full stretch. Stand up using your legs to get yourself into the top position before lowering yourself to the bottom. Repeat until you are unable to safely control the downward movement of your body.

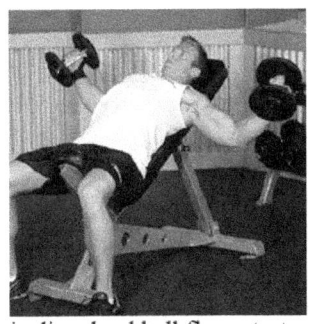 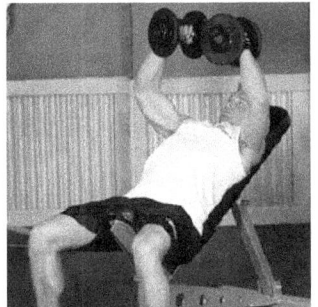

incline dumbbell flyes-start   finish

Chest Routine #3
Push-ups- 1 set to failure
Using rotational push-up handles space your hands slightly wider than shoulder width. Lower yourself down to the bottom position, pause one second, then press yourself up to the point just prior to lockout. As you become stronger you may need to add weight by having your partner add a weight plate to your back.
No rest
Barbell bench press- 1 set of 8 reps to failure plus 4 forced negatives at the end of the set
Bring the bar slowly to a point and inch or two above the nipples, pause for a second then press to the point just prior to lockout. Do not rest the bar on your chest at any time. After completing the standard reps press the bar up and have your training partner apply extra pressure to the bar as you resist the downward motion to a count of 8. After doing four of these reps you should have exhausted your muscles.
Cable crossovers- 1 set of 12 reps to failure
Grab both handles of a crossover machine and bring them in front of you in an arc motion. Pause for one second then return to the starting position. Squeeze your pec muscles at the point where the handles come together for an increased effect.

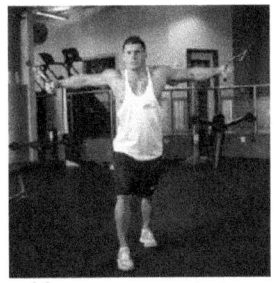 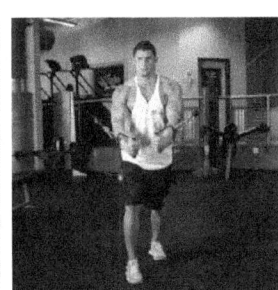

cable crossovers-start   finish

Back

Back Routine #1
Nautilus or other comparable machine pullovers- 1 set of 15 reps to failure
Sit in the machine and fasten the seat belt if provided. Place your elbows against the pads and gently rest your hands against the bar. Let the movement arm back as far as is comfortable being sure not to overextend your arms and shoulder girdle. Inhale deeply as you go back. Exhale as you bring your arms forward and down in front of you. Pause for one second then return to the stretched position. Repeat.

Machine or dumbbell rows- 1 set of 12 reps to failure
Using either a machine or a pair of dumbbells extend your arms and get a good stretch as you inhale deeply. Pull the dumbbells or movement arm in toward your chest, pause one second while squeezing your back muscles and lower back to the start position.

Medium grip cable pulldowns- 1 set of 8 reps to failure plus 4 forced reps at the end of the set
Using a medium grip, preferably with a bar made so your palms face each other, let the weight pull your hands up over your head for a full stretch. Isolating the effort mostly to your back muscles, pull the bar down to your abdominal area. Pause for one second then return to the start position to repeat for a total of 8 reps. Squeeze your back muscles hard while at the fully contracted position for more effect. Have your partner give just enough assistance to allow you to complete an additional 4 forced reps.

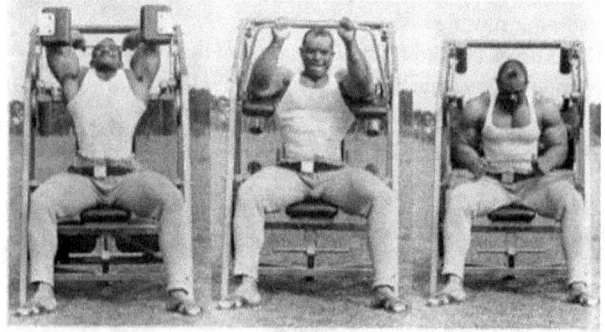

Nautilus machine pullover-start, mid-point and finish
The great Sergio Oliva demonstrating the exercise

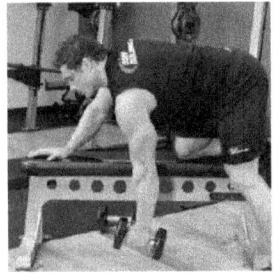 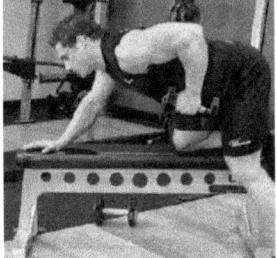

one-arm dumbbell row-start   finish

Back Routine #2
Partial rep medium grip cable pulldowns- 1 set of 12 reps
Divide a pulldown movement into three distinct zones, the first third, the next third and the final third zone. After getting a good stretch at the top, pull the bar down stopping one third of the way before returning to the top position. Complete a total of 4 reps in this zone before moving on to the next two zones and training them in the same way.

Barbell rows- 1 set of 8, 10-second static holds
You should be using weights that allow you to hold the bar in position for 10 seconds only. Pull the barbell up until at the top of the lift, which is the point of maximum contraction. Hold for 10 seconds before setting the barbell down. Rest 10 seconds then repeat. It will be necessary to reduce the weight as you progress or else it will be impossible to hold the weight for 10 seconds. This is a very effective method of training but it takes practice to perfect the amount of weight to use throughout the exercise.

Seated reverse flyes- 1 set of 10 reps plus 4 pure negative reps
Sit backward in a pek dek machine or in a rear delt machine. Grab the handles and extend your arms backward as if you were a bird flapping its wings in a reverse motion. Pause for one second then return to the start position. After completing 10 reps have your partner do all of the lifting of the weight and transfer the resistance to you so you can lower the weight using an eight count. Repeat for an additional 3 reps. Ending the set in this fashion works the muscle much harder than if you had ended the set after the traditional reps.

Back routine #3
Barbell rows- 1 set of 8 reps rest-pause style
Load a barbell with your 90 1RM (90% of the maximum you can lift for one rep). Lift the weight to your chest while bending over the bar horizontal to the floor. Pause for one second then return the bar to the floor. Stand up and breathe deeply while resting for 10 seconds. Repeat for a total of 8, single maximum reps. Note: you will need to reduce the poundage as you progress in the set.

Stiff-arm pulldowns on cable machine- 1 set of 12 reps, omni-contraction style

Attach a medium length straight bar to the upper pulley on a cable machine. Keeping your arms locked in a straight position pull the bar straight down until it touches your knees. Pause for one second before letting the bar up $1/3^{rd}$ of the way. Stop for one second before proceeding to mid-point. Pause for one second then continue until the bar is just before the start position. Pause for one second and return to the start position. At each stop you should attempt to reverse the direction of the bar but if the proper amount of weight is loaded you will be unable to.

Machine pullovers- 1 set of 10 reps, max holds

Load the weight heavy enough to allow 20 second holds. Place your elbows on the pads and bring the movement arm to the point of maximum contraction, which is three quarters of the way through the range of motion. Hold the movement arms for 20 seconds then return to the start position. Repeat after resting for 10 seconds. Do a total of 10 holds.

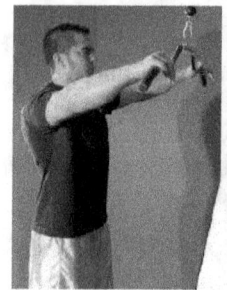 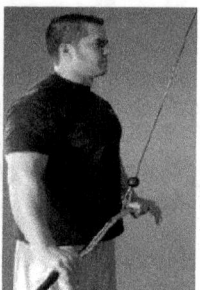

stiff-arm pulldown-start   finish

This workout uses three different advanced high intensity techniques, rest-pause during the barbell rows, omni-contraction with the stiff-arm pulldowns and max holds during the pullovers. Rest-pause is an excellent technique that results in the trainee being able to maximize his/her efforts without having to cease training due to the common burning sensation that results from training hard. This is avoided because the lactic acid is flushed out during the 10-second rest between reps.

Omni-contraction increases the intensity of effort by having the trainee perform three different holds during the negative phase of the movement.

Max holds, or super holds, subject the muscles to maximum contractions during the 20 second holds. This is similar to isometric contraction holds.

Shoulders

Shoulder routine #1
Seated lateral raises on machine or with dumbbells - 1 set of 12 reps+ burn reps

Select a weight that allows you to complete 12 reps to failure. Place your hands against the pads and extend the movement arms up until you reach the end position parallel with the floor. Pause for one second then return to the beginning position. After you reach muscular exhaustion and are unable to get another full rep, do as many burns, or partial reps until you are unable to move the handles at all.

This completely exhausts the muscle and causes a deep burn hence the name burn reps. This burn, it has been shown in studies, causes a release of human growth hormone, a very important hormone that is responsible for both fat loss and muscle gain. This movement can be done with a pair of dumbbells as noted. To use dumbbells, sit or stand while holding a dumbbell in each hand. Keeping a small bend in your arms bring the weights up from your sides until they're parallel with the floor. This is a side lateral raise movement.

Front lateral raises- 1 set of 12 reps

Begin the movement with dumbbells held at your thighs in the front. Keeping a small bend in your arms lift the weights to a position slightly above shoulder level. Lower the weights under control.

Machine presses- 1 set of 8 reps+ 6 negative-only reps at the end of the set

After selecting a weight that causes muscular exhaustion at 8 reps lift the handles to a position just prior to lockout. Pause for one second then return to the start position. After the 8th rep have a partner lift the handles to the top then transition the resistance to you using a smooth change. Lower the weight to a count of 8 then repeat.

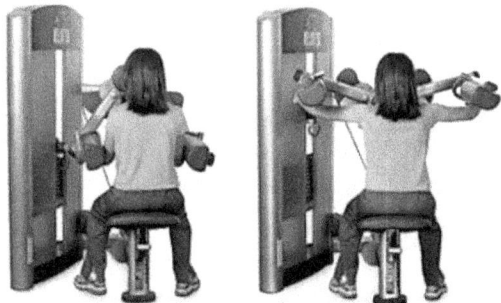

machine lateral raise-start and finish

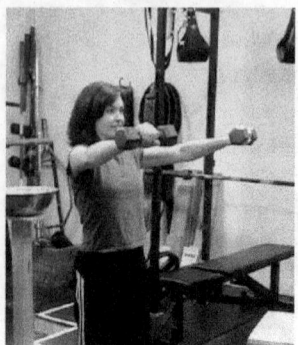
dumbbell front raise-finish

Shoulder routine #2
Bent-over raises- 1 set of 12 reps + burn reps
Bend forward until perpendicular to the floor. Grab two dumbbells and while keeping a small bend in your arms, lift the weights up and out to the side until they are parallel to the floor. Pause one second then repeat. After the 12 reps are finished do a series of small, partial burn reps until you are unable to move the weights.

Standing Barbell Presses- 1 set of 10 reps + 4 forced reps
Load a barbell with a weight that allows you to complete 10 reps. Clean the weight and do 10 reps. Have a partner provide enough assistance to allow you to complete an additional 4 reps.

Seated barbell presses in a power rack- 1 set of 12 reps
Set the pins in the power rack so the range of motion starts at the beginning of the press and the bar stops at the second set of pins one third of the way through the movement. Do 4 reps in this zone. At the end of the 4th rep press the bar against the pins with all your strength for 10 seconds then release. Reset the pins so the bar begins at the end of the 1st zone and ends at ¾ of the press motion. Do 4 reps pressing on the pins with the bar for 10 seconds. Reset the pins and complete 4 reps in the final zone in the same fashion as the first two zones.

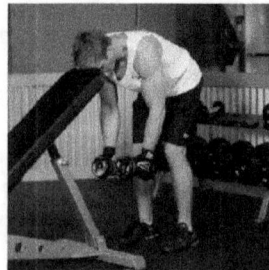
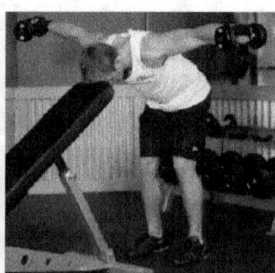
bent-over lateral raises-start   finish

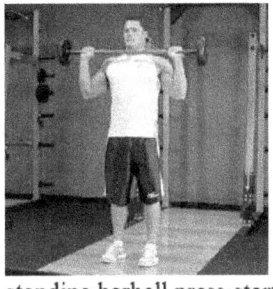 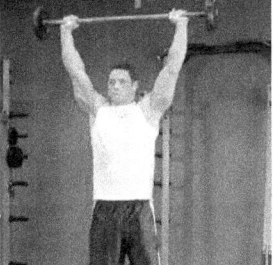

standing barbell press-start   finish

Shoulder routine #3
Standing dumbbell presses- up and down the rack
Begin the medium heavy dumbbells and do 8 reps. Grab the next pair and
lift for 8 reps. Continue up the rack until you max out with a pair of
dumbbells to muscular failure. Work your way back down the stack until
reaching muscular exhaustion.
Machine seated laterals- 1 set of 12, 10-second holds
Select a weight that is heavy for a 10-second hold but not maximum
resistance. Hold the handles of the machine at the finish position just prior to
lockout for 10 seconds. Rest 10 seconds, select the next heaviest weight and
perform a 10-second hold. Continue increasing the weight and doing 10-
second holds until you reach the point of barely being able to maintain a 10-
second hold. Begin decreasing the weight and doing 10-second holds while
working your way down the stack.

Biceps

Bicep routine #1
Incline dumbbell curls- 1 set of 12 reps
Using a weight that causes muscular exhaustion at 12 reps curl the
dumbbells deliberately with no momentum or swing. Lower the weight to a
count of six. Pause one second at the bottom before performing the next rep.
Palms-facing pulldowns on cable machine- 1 set of 12 reps+ 4 forced reps
Use a straight bar that attaches to a cable machine. Select a resistance that
allows 12 reps only. Using a shoulder-width grip with palms facing you, pull
the bar down to your upper chest, pause for one second then return to the
beginning. After completing 12 reps have your partner apply just enough
assistance to allow you to complete an additional 4 reps.
After you gain some experience with this exercise you will be able to relax
your back muscles and focus the majority of the effort on the biceps
muscles, making this exercise much more effective for biceps training.

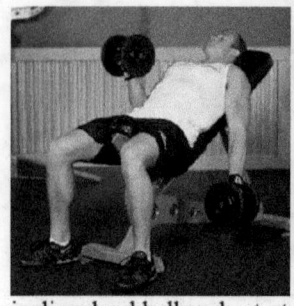 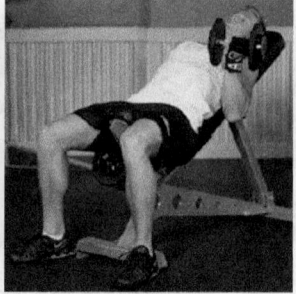

incline dumbbell curls-start   finish

Bicep routine #2
Barbell curls- 1 set of 12 reps rest-pause style
Load a barbell with enough weight to allow one maximum rep. Lift the bar using no momentum to the top, pause one second then lower to a count of 4. Set the bar down and rest for 10 seconds. Repeat for 11 more reps. It will be necessary to reduce the weight as you progress through the set to allow you to complete each rep. It is very important to use good form throughout the set to keep the tension on the muscle.

Behind-head rope curls- 1 set of 12 reps + 5 static holds
Sit on the seat facing the cable after attaching a rope handle to the high pulley. Grab a rope in each hand and curl them back alongside your head. Hold the rope there for several seconds to get a strong contraction before returning to the start position. After finishing the set perform 5, 10-second static holds with 5 seconds rest between each.

Bicep routine #3
Dumbbell concentration curls- 1 set of 10 reps +3 forced reps
You can use either a standing, bent-over position with your elbow fixed on your knee or a seated position for this exercise. To do the seated version grab a dumbbell and while sitting, curl the dumbbell up to your shoulder. Pause for one second then return to the beginning position. During the exercise your elbow should be fixed on your leg located on the same side as the arm that is being trained. After 10 reps use your other hand to assist in completion of 3 additional reps. Switch hands and train the other side in the same way.

Curl machine- 1 set of 12 partial reps
Use a Nautilus or similar curl machine for this exercise. Select a weight that causes muscular exhaustion at 12 reps. Begin by curling the arms one third of the way up and hold for one second at the top of the partial rep. Complete four reps in this zone before doing an additional four reps in the middle zone. Finish by completing four reps in the top zone.

Triceps

Triceps routine #1
Standing triceps pushdowns- 1 set of 10 reps + 4 forced reps
Standing with your legs shoulder width apart lock your elbows at your sides. Begin with the triceps rope or triceps handle in front of your face and push the handle straight down in front of you until it is fully extended. Pause for one second then return to the start position. After completing 10 reps have your partner assist you with just enough pressure to enable you to complete an additional 4 reps.

Close-grip bench presses- 1 set of 12 reps rest-pause style
You can use either a barbell or bench press machine for this one. Use a grip that is approximately 12 inches apart. Press the weight like you would a normal bench press. Using a maximum weight press the weight for one rep, avoiding lockout. Rest 10 seconds then repeat. It will be necessary to reduce the weight as you progress through the set to allow you to complete the reps.

Triceps routine #2
Triceps kickbacks- 1 set of 12 holds
Use dumbbells that cause maximum effort during a 15 second hold. Do a set of 12 holds with a 10-second rest in between. As you progress through the set you will need to reduce the weight to allow you to complete the set. To do this exercise, lean forward while holding a dumbbell in each hand. Press both dumbbells all the way back until you are unable to push them back any further.

Triceps machine dips- 1 set of 10 reps omni-contraction style
Sit upright in the dip machine. Press the movement arms down to just before lockout. Pause for one second before beginning the negative portion of the movement. Stop the motion one third of the way and hold for five seconds. Lower an additional third and hold another five seconds. Finish by lowering near the finish point and hold for a final five seconds. Repeat for 10 reps.

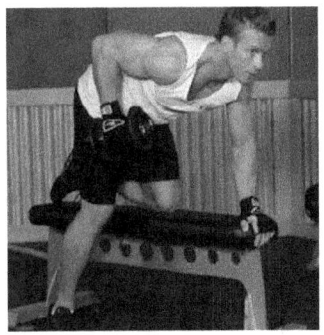
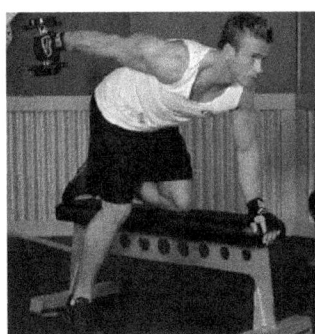

tricep kickback-start   finish

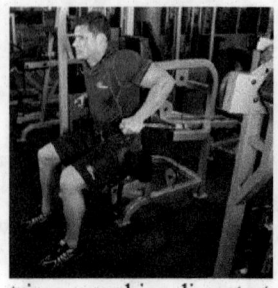
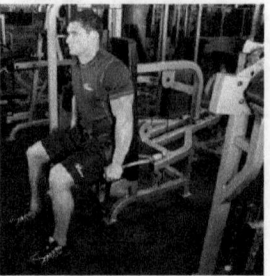

triceps machine dips-start   finish

Triceps routine #3

Two-hand overhead triceps dumbbell extensions - 1 set of 12 reps omni-contraction style

Grab a dumbbell with two hands and hold it behind your head. Lock your elbows at the side of your head and extend the dumbbell straight overhead. Lower the dumbbell-stopping one third of the way and hold the dumbbell for 10 seconds. Lower to mid-point and hold for 10 seconds. Finish the rep by lowering to the point just prior to the bottom and hold for 10 seconds. Repeat for a total of 12 reps.

Triceps machine dips- 1 set of 12 holds pyramid style

After selecting a heavy weight begin by holding the movement arms of the dip machine for 10 seconds at the point just prior to lockout. Lower the weight back to the stack and rest for 5 seconds. For the second hold use a weight that is heavier than the first hold. Work your way up in weight until you hit a peak weight that barely allows you to hold the movement arms of the machine for 10 seconds. Work your way down in weight until you bottom out at the 12th hold. This is a great way to work up in resistance and work your way back down as your muscles become exhausted.

The principles behind these HIT routines

As you quickly noticed, the routines outlined above use an abbreviated workout time coupled with intense efforts using non-traditional training variables such as static holds, omni-contraction, rest-pause, forced reps and negative reps among others. These techniques, or variables, form a system that is scientifically based to produce rapid gains in muscle size and strength.

Since we are bodybuilding with this program, and not powerlifting, we are concerned less with the amount of weight lifted and more with focusing the resistance on the muscle(s) being trained. To grow muscle we need to give it the proper amount of stimulus using a protocol that uses the correct amount of reps, sets and time under tension so we can avoid over training and maximize muscle growth. After training the muscles correctly we need to rest, rest, rest! Remember, muscle growth is stimulated by training but occurs during rest.

The HIT variables are designed to dramatically increase the intensity of effort. This shocks the muscles into new growth. Intensity is often described incorrectly as the amount of weight one can lift but is actually measured by the amount of effort put forth while training. Another false statement states that it is possible to increase training intensity by upping the number of sets performed for a body part. There is a scientifically proven ratio that states that the higher the intensity of effort the lower the set count must be and vice versa.

The original Nautilus high intensity routines as espoused by Nautilus inventor Arthur Jones were based on a three-day per week total body workout. This program produced good gains in strength and conditioning but had shortcomings. The problem was that in order to properly focus maximum effort on a muscle group it is necessary to have abundant energy, which isn't possible while using a full body workout program. The best way to give optimum effort to each muscle group is to use a slit routine such as:

Monday-legs, abdominals
Wednesday-chest, shoulders
Friday-back, arms

There are many variations of this and you may wish to alter your schedule to allow extra focus on one particular muscle group that may be lagging behind the others.

Proper amount of sets per muscle group

Once you are accustomed to training on a regular basis and have become more advanced in your training you need to be sure that you are using the correct rep count, time under tension and sets. For larger muscle groups such as legs, back and chest three max intensity sets should be optimal. For smaller muscle groups such as shoulders, biceps and triceps two sets are ideal. Notice how I said max intensity. This means that each set must be done with all-out effort, which is never easy. Each set must contain one or two high intensity variables to make it effective at this low set count.

Frequency of training

The number of times that you train a particular muscle group during a set period of time is very important. If excessive amount of training is done you will experience the negative effects such as muscle size loss, decrease of strength and overall feeling of fatigue leading to a disinterest in training.

A factor in determining the frequency of training is the ability of the trainee to recuperate from a given workout session. Some people recover from training much more rapidly than others. As you become more experienced you will quickly be able to determine if you recover more rapidly or need additional rest days before resuming training for the same muscle group.

It is very important to allow your entire body systems ample time to recuperate or you will be unable to make gains. A good rule of thumb is to train each muscle group once every seven days and decrease that to once every ten days if you haven't made a full recovery. As you become stronger it will be necessary to reduce the volume of work and frequency of training because you will be subjecting yourself to more extreme demands due to your increased muscle strength.

Variable Intensity Training Routines

This type of training is a close cousin to HIT training. Instead of taking each set of an exercise to muscular exhaustion we take some sets to one to two reps short of failure while taking others to muscular exhaustion. We continue to follow the principle of intensity relative to volume. That principle states that the higher the amount of work performed or volume (sets) the lower the intensity must be. It is very important to keep the number of sets within a logical framework and not resort to the "more is better" philosophy that many bodybuilders and weight trainees have adopted.

Benefits of training with the variable intensity approach

After a time of using the HIT approach in your workouts your body will be accustomed to the all-out effort you are putting forth in your training and the results you have been getting from your training will slow down. The variable intensity approach allows you to disrupt homeostasis and get your body systems "guessing" again. When this happens you will begin experiencing new progress in conditioning, strength and muscle size increase.

While the HIT protocol is much safer to use than traditional types of training since it uses controlled movement as opposed to momentum and loose form in exercises, it is beneficial to lower the intensity at times to give yourself an emotional and physical break from constantly driving yourself to muscular failure.

The following workout routines present programs that will get you great results whether you are looking for increased strength, muscle growth or better overall conditioning. We will be using some of the same techniques that we used during the HIT sessions to keep the intensity fairly high because that is what results in new gains.

Legs

Routine #1
Leg extensions- 1 set of 15 reps
Sit in the machine and extend your legs upward until you reach the top extended position. Hold at maximum contraction for three seconds then return to the start position. Do all reps in a controlled fashion using a weight that enables you to terminate the set one rep before muscular exhaustion.
Barbell squats- 1 set of 12 reps
Use a power rack or smith machine if you are training alone otherwise a good squat rack and training partner will work well. While doing this exercise look up straight ahead and keep your back straight to avoid injury. By the 12th rep you should be near muscular exhaustion.
Leg lunges- 1 set of 12 reps each leg
Hold a pair of dumbbells, one in each hand. Step forward with your left leg straight out in front of you. Use a deep step and bend down until your leg is parallel to the floor. Push yourself back with your outstretched leg and repeat with your right leg. Complete the rest of the set in this fashion.
Leg presses-1 set of 15 reps
Load the machine with a weight that causes muscular exhaustion at 15 reps. Set the machine so you get a full leg movement. Bring the weight back until your knees almost touch your chest. Pause for one second then press the footplate until you are one inch from lockout. Repeat for another 14 reps.
Leg curls-2 sets of 15 reps
Select a weight that finishes each set one rep from failure. Place the foam pad midway between your ankles and calf muscles. Curl the weight up as far as you can and squeeze your hamstring muscles hard at the top of the movement. Pause one second then return to the start position. Repeat for a total of 15 reps. Rest one minute then do a second set using a weight that is 25% lighter than the first set.
Standing calf raises- 1 set of 15 reps
Select a weight that stops one rep shy of failure. Get a great stretch at the bottom of the movement by keeping your legs in the fully extended position with knees locked and lower all the way down as far as you can go. Extend your feet up on the balls of your feet and tense the calf muscles at the top of the movement.
Donkey calf raises- 1 set of 12 reps. Use a machine or have someone sit on your back while you are bent forward, parallel to the floor. Support yourself

by placing your elbows on a bench if not using a machine. Get a full stretch by lowering your heels as close to the floor as you can before pressing your heels up to full extension.

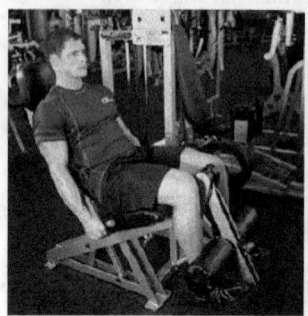 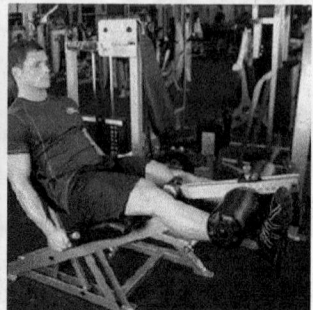

leg extensions-start   finish

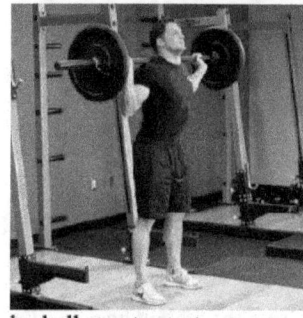 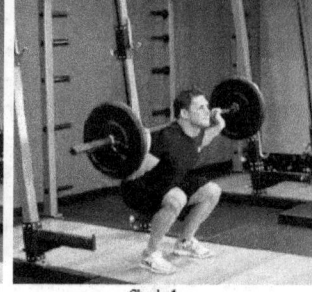

barbell squats-start   finish

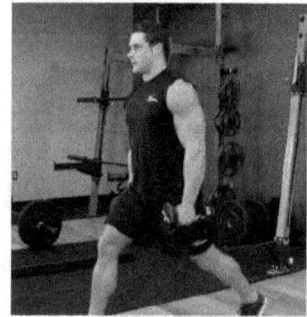 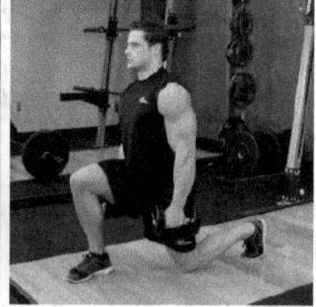

leg lunges-start   finish

Leg lunges enable the trainee to focus all effort on the one leg being trained and resembles an outstretched squat movement. The deep step out in front multiplies the intensity of effort on the leg muscles. Both the front of the leg and the hamstrings are trained in this exercise.

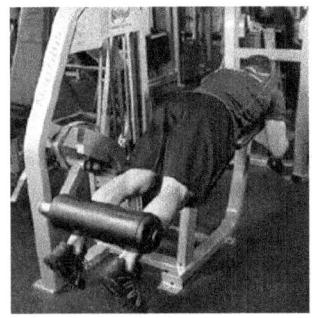 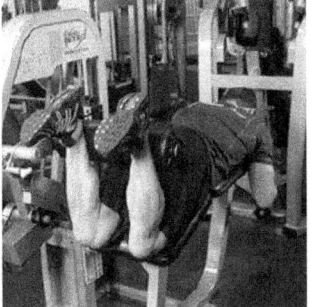

lying leg curls-start   finish

Routine #2
Dumbbell squats- 1 set of 15 reps
Holding a dumbbell in each hand, lower yourself down into a deep squat position. Keeping your head up and your back straight, push yourself up to the top position of the squat. Repeat until one rep before failure. These are great if you are training alone and don't have someone to spot you or you have lower back issues that may be aggravated by squats. They also alleviate the feeling of holding a heavy weight on your shoulders and allow you to really focus the effort on your leg muscles. This exercise trains your frontal thigh muscles but if you descend down low you will also be working your hamstring muscles.

Stiff-legged deadlifts- 1 set of 12 reps
Grab a pair of dumbbells, and while keeping your knees locked, lean forward lowering the dumbbells to the floor. Lift the weights in a deadlift motion until you are standing erect. You should end the set one rep short of failure. Be careful with the amount of weight you are lifting with this exercise or you will risk a lower back or hamstring injury. Throughout the movement use a smooth, steady motion with absolutely no momentum. This exercise trains your hamstring muscles.

Dumbbell squats- 1 set of 10 reps
Do a second set consisting of 10 reps performed the same way as the first set except this time take the set to failure.

Inner/outer thigh-hip flexor- 1 set of 15 reps
Various manufacturers make machines to train the inner and outer thighs and hip flexor muscles. This exercise builds strong hip muscles as well as the inner and outer thighs. This is an area that is often overlooked but is very important to leg strength and development nevertheless.

Seated calf raises- 2 sets of 15 reps to failure
Sit in a calf machine or hold a weight plate on your lap. Your legs should be bent and your upper legs should be parallel to the floor. Place the balls of your feet on a block of wood if not using a machine. Lower your heels to the floor for a full stretch. Extend your feet up on the balls of your feet until you

extend them up fully. Tense your calves hard at the top. Repeat for 14 additional reps. Rest one minute then perform the second set.

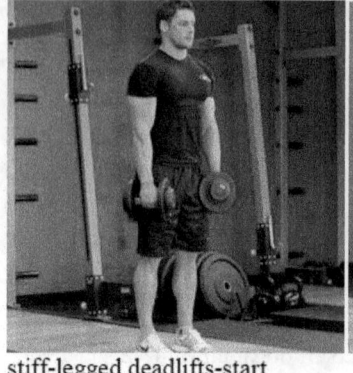 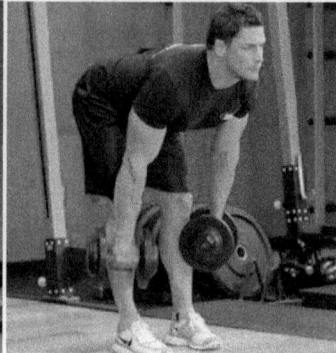

stiff-legged deadlifts-start   finish

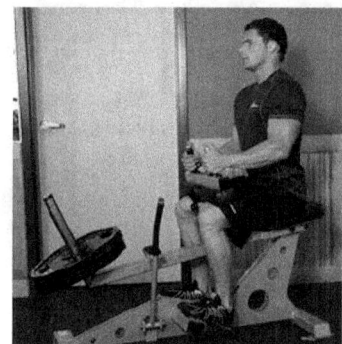 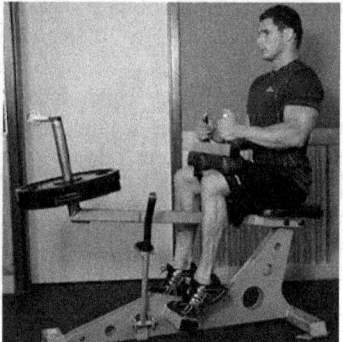

seated calf raises-start   finish

Routine #3

Leg presses- 1 set of 100 reps
Select a weight that allows 10 reps, stopping one rep before failure. Rest 10 seconds then do a second set of 10 reps after lowering the weight. Continue in this fashion until you complete a total of 100 reps. This set will give you a great pump. Research has shown that training such as this leads to an increase in the release of human growth hormone, one of the most important hormones in the growth of muscle mass and strength.

Leg extensions- 1 set of 100 reps
Perform this exercise in exactly the same fashion as the leg presses. Make sure to flex your leg muscles hard for 3 seconds at the full extension of this movement.

Leg curls- 2 sets of 12 reps each
Do both sets stopping one rep short of failure. Rest one minute between sets.

Standing calf raises- 2 sets of 15 reps

Do the first set to failure; rest one minute then do the second set finishing one rep short of failure as well.

Chest

Routine #1
Dumbbell bench presses- 1 set up and down the rack

Begin with a moderately heavy pair of dumbbells and do 10 reps in the flat bench press. Rest 10 seconds then move up to the next heavier set of dumbbells and do 10 reps with those. Keep repeating this by moving up in weight until you are unable to get a minimum of 6 reps. Move down the rack of dumbbells in the same fashion that you moved up until you work your way down to a moderate weight set. Every set should be to muscular exhaustion.

Cable crossovers high position-1set of 12 reps

Get a good stretch at the beginning of this exercise by bringing your arms as far back as possible. Using a downward arc motion bring the handles to your thighs before crossing them in front of you. Pause for one second then repeat. Finish the set at 12 reps stopping one rep shy of failure.

Cable crossovers low position- 1 set of 12 reps

Do the exercise same as above but set the pulleys low on the machine. With this setting you will raise the handles in an upward arc until they are in front of you at head level.

End the set one rep shy of failure.

Pushups- 1 set to failure

Space your hands slightly wider than shoulder width. Lower yourself until you are almost touching the floor, pause for one second then press yourself up. Continue until you hit failure.

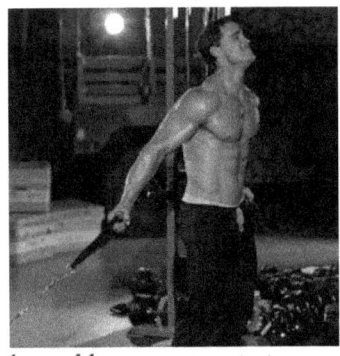
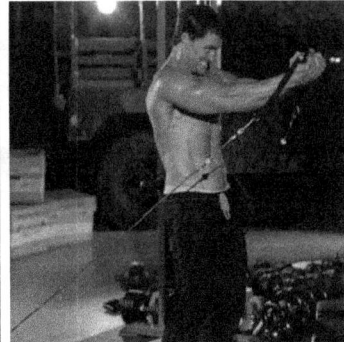

low cable crossovers-start   finish

Routine #2
Decline dumbbell flyes- 1 set of 12 reps

Use dumbbells that allow you to finish the set one rep prior to failure. Lie on a decline bench and lower the dumbbells for a full stretch. Curl them up in an arc until they just touch; pause one second then return to the start position. Repeat for a total of 12 reps.

Machine bench press- 1 set of 12 holds
Load the machine with a heavy weight that allows you to only raise the weight stack ½-1". Lift the weight off the stack and hold it for 10 seconds. Rest for 10 seconds then repeat with a weight that is 10 lbs lighter. Continue working down the stack until you complete the 12th hold. This is a maximum effort set so use as heavy a weight as possible for each hold.

Incline machine bench press- Multiple sets totaling 100 reps
Select a weight that allows you to complete 10 reps, ending the set one rep prior to failure. After doing the first set lower the weight then repeat for another set of 10 reps. Continue until you complete a total of 100 reps, which should be ten total sets. After this set you should have a great pump and an intense burn in the muscle.

Machine dips- 2 sets of 10 partial reps
Select a weight that allows you to complete 10 reps, going one rep shy of failure. Press the machine arms down one third of the way and return to the start position. Repeat this for several additional partial reps. Press the arms down in the next zone at mid-point and do several more reps. Finish the set by doing the remaining reps in the last third zone. For the second set complete it the same as the first except take it to muscular failure on the final rep.

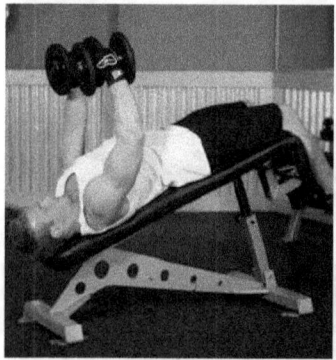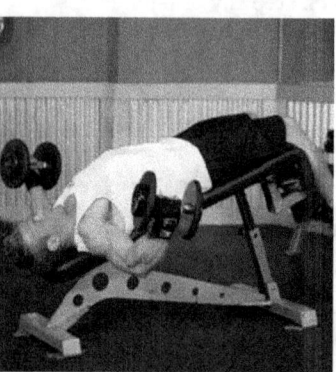

decline dumbbell flyes-start   finish

Decline dumbbell flyes and decline bench presses train the entire pectoral muscles but focus additional stress on the bottom portion of the pec. While it is impossible to "shape" a muscle, this exercise will ensure that your lower pec development is even with the rest of the chest muscles.

44

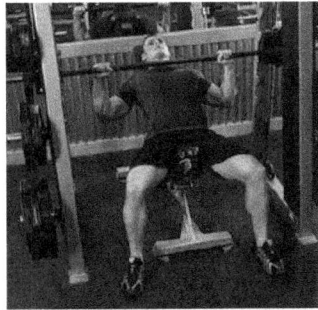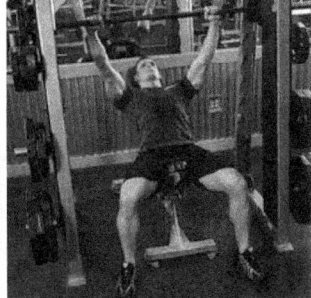

incline bench presses in smith machine-start   finish

Routine #3
Pek Dek or machine flyes- 2 sets of 12 reps
Select a weight that allows you to finish 12 reps, stopping one rep short of failure. After completing that set rest for 30 seconds. For the second set select a weight that brings you to failure at the 12th rep. It is very important to use good form and get a really good stretch at the beginning of the movement before bringing the movement arms in front of you for a full contraction. This prepares your chest muscles for a more intense contraction, which causes more muscle fibers to be used during the exercise, causing more growth stimulation.

Dumbbell bench presses- 1 set of 12 reps omni-contraction
Press the dumbbells up stopping before lockout. Pause for one second then lower them 1/3rd of the way and hold for five seconds. Lower them to the mid-point and hold for five seconds then complete the rep by holding the weights for five seconds at the beginning position. Repeat the last 11 reps in the same fashion.

Machine dips- 2 sets, 12 reps first one, heavy partials in the second set
For your first set do 12 reps in the standard fashion, ending the set one rep shy of failure. Your second set should be a maximum effort set. Select a heavy weight that allows you to lift the weight off the stack only an inch or two. Repeat for 6 reps, the final rep ending in muscular exhaustion.

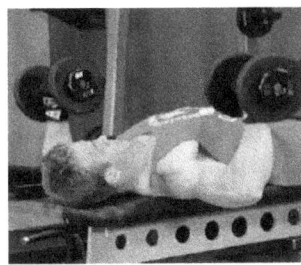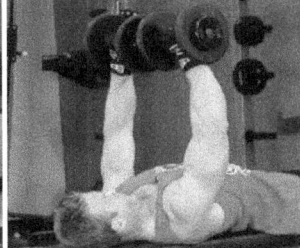

dumbbell bench press-start   finish

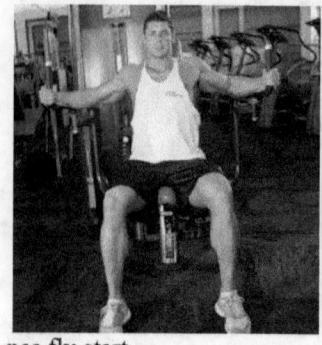 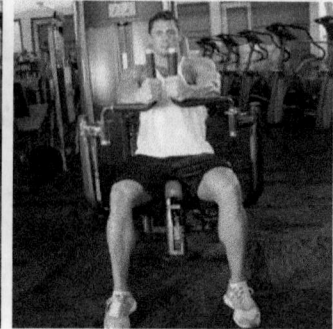

pec fly-start   finish

Back

Routine #1
Dumbbell rows- 1 set of 12 reps
This exercise can be done by rowing either one or two dumbbells at a time. The advantage of using one is the ability to support your back with your free hand to prevent a back injury. It is also great for getting extra range of motion and concentrating all of your effort into training one side of your back at a time. Stop the set one rep shy of failure.
Dumbbell or machine pullovers- 1 set of 15 reps
Use one dumbbell or a pullover machine for this movement. If using a dumbbell sit on the floor and arch your back over a bench. Holding the dumbbell overhead, breathe deeply, and with bent arms lower the dumbbell back over the bench. Pause one second then return to the beginning position as you exhale. Stop the set one rep short of failure.
Seated cable pulldowns- 2 sets of 10 reps
Both of these sets should be to failure with as heavy a weight as you can handle for 10 reps. Use a grip that is approximately 18-24" apart with the palms of your hands facing each other. Get a good stretch at the beginning of this exercise and pull the bar down to your lower chest area as you exhale. Pause for one second then repeat for another 9 reps.
Rest one minute between sets.

Routine #2
Machine pullovers- 1 set of 12 static holds
Select a weight that allows maximum exertion while doing a 20 second hold. Work your way up the weight stack performing the holds until you hit your maximum weight that you can handle then work your way back down the stack, achieving a total of 12 holds.
Rest should be 10 seconds between holds. This allows time for your body to flush lactic acid out of your muscles and prevent you from ending the set

prematurely due to lactic acid buildup or being winded. This is a great isolation exercise that uses your back muscles to perform almost all of the work. Once we exhaust your back muscles with this exercise we are able to push them even further past failure with the next exercise, which is a compound one.

Barbell rows- 2 sets of 10 reps

Complete a set of barbell rows with a weight heavy enough to take your muscles to the point of failure on the 10th rep. After setting the barbell down, reduce the weight 30% and do the second set to failure with 10 reps. Rest one minute then proceed to the final exercise.

Ab strap pulldowns- 1 sets of 12 reps, 1 set of 15 reps

Hook a good pair of ab straps to a high pulley attachment on a cable machine. Place both arms in the straps so the entire upper arm is in a horizontal position in the straps. Extend your arms up to get a good stretch and bring them down to your side and tense your lats hard. Finish the set by completing 12 reps just shy of failure. Rest one minute then repeat for 15 reps to failure. This exercise is great because it converts a traditionally compound exercise into an isolation one by taking most of the arm effort out of the exercise by using the ab straps.

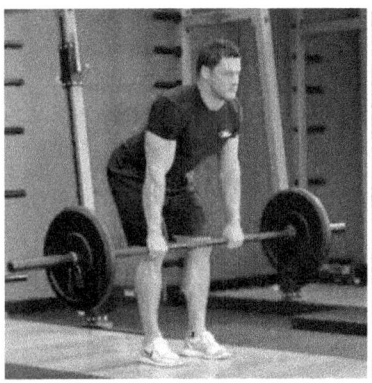 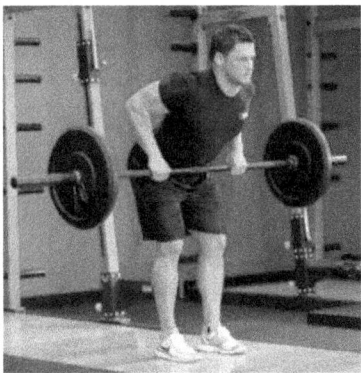

barbell row-start   finish

Routine #3

Power rack partial deadlifts- 1 set of 10 reps

Set the pins on the power rack so the barbell sits in the rack 18 inches off the floor. Load it with a heavy weight that will cause muscular failure at 10 reps. Deadlift the bar up all the way to a full deadlift. Lower the bar back to the pins but don't set it down. Repeat for a total of 10 reps. The advantage of this exercise is it eliminates the weak link in the deadlift by beginning the movement at an 18" height instead of off the floor. By avoiding the weak "sticking point" you are able to concentrate on the stronger portion allowing you to build more strength and size by using a heavier weight than you could use if you did a full deadlifting movement.

Palms-up two-handed rope pull- 1 set of 12 reps

Grab the rope handle with a palms-up grip. Pull the rope into your upper abdomen and squeeze your lats hard before returning to the beginning. The hand position in this exercise enables you to use your biceps muscle to assist your back in pulling the rope. Remember that you must allow your back muscles to do most of the pulling. The way to do this is to focus your concentration on your back muscles while relaxing your biceps as much as you can. Of course you will have to have enough tension in your biceps to allow you to pull the weight. Finish this set one rep shy of failure.

Machine pullovers- 1 set of 12 static holds

Use a maximum weight to cause you to struggle to hold the movement arms for 10 seconds in each of these holds. Begin at your maximum weight holding it for 10 seconds before returning the weight to the stack. Rest 10 seconds, then after reducing the weight a plate or two, do another 10 second hold. Continue until you have worked your way down the stack, hitting your 12th hold. Perform your holds at different zones in the movement to hit your back from different angles.

Seated reverse back flyes- 2 sets of 12 reps

Select a weight that enables you to end the set one rep shy of failure at 12 reps. Either use a reverse flye machine or a chest pek dek or flye machine. Sit into the machine facing the back pad and grab the handles. Make sure your arms are bent slightly and bring the handles backward until they are horizontal out to your sides. Pause one second then return the handles to the start position, repeating for a total of 12 reps. Rest one minute then do the second set in the same fashion as the first.

Shoulders

Routine #1

Seated machine laterals- 2 sets of 12 reps

Select a weight that allows you to end the set one rep shy of failure at 12 reps. Sit in the machine and place your hands and arms against the pads on each of the arms. Using a smooth motion raise your arms up until they are parallel with the floor. Pause one second then return to the start position. Rest one minute then complete the second set of 12 reps, stopping one rep short of failure.

Machine presses- 1 set of 10 reps

Select a weight that causes failure at 10 reps. Press the arms up to the position just prior to lockout. Pause one second then return to the start position. Repeat for a total of 10 reps.

Routine #2
Barbell presses- 1 set of 12 reps
While standing press a barbell overhead to the position prior to lockout. Pause one second then lower the bar. Repeat for a total of 12 reps. Go to failure on this set.
Front lateral raises- 1 set of 12 reps
Grab a pair of dumbbells and using a steady motion, lift them in front of you until they are slightly above shoulder height. Pause one second then return them to the start position. Repeat for a total of 12 reps. End the set one rep short of failure.
Bent over lateral raises- 1 set of 12 reps
Grab a pair of dumbbells and bend over until your torso is parallel with the floor. Keep your arms slightly bent and raise your arms until they are parallel with the floor. Pause one second then return to the start position, stopping one rep short of failure. Use a smooth motion with this exercise being mindful not to use any momentum or jerking.
Side lateral raises- 1 set of 12 reps
Stand erect with a dumbbell in each hand at your side. With your arms slightly bent, lift the dumbbells out to each side until they are slightly above shoulder level. Pause for one second then return them to the beginning position.

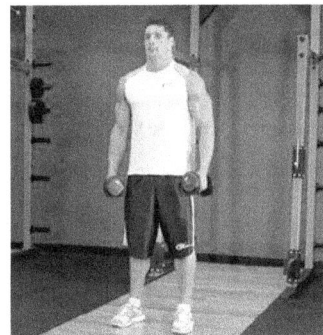 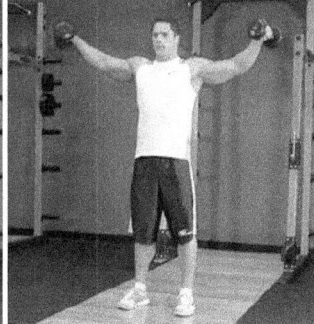

side lateral raises-start   finish

Routine #3
Dumbbell presses up and down the rack- multiple sets
Grab two dumbbells and do a set of standing dumbbell presses. These can be completed by pressing both weights up at the same time or alternating presses one arm at a time. All of these sets should be carried to one rep short of failure. After finishing the first set grab the next heaviest pair and do a set of presses in the same way with them. Continue going up the rack until you peak at the heaviest set you can handle. Work your way back down the rack until the weights become too light.

Seated press behind neck- 1 set of 12 reps rest pause
Use a machine preferably for this exercise. Select a weight that allows only a
one-rep max. Lift the handles up using a smooth motion stopping prior to
lockout. Return the weight to the stack and rest for 10 seconds before
reducing the weight and doing a second rep. Continue until a total of 12 reps
are completed

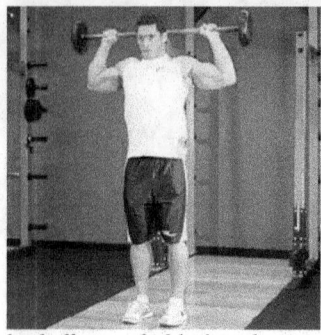 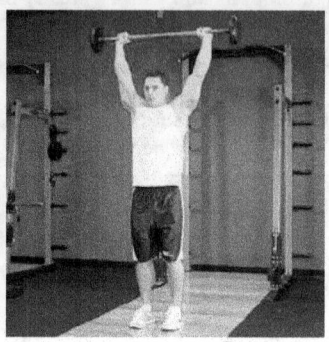

barbell press behind neck-start   finish

Arms

Routine #1
Barbell curls- 2 sets of 10 reps
Load the bar with a weight that allows 10 reps without going to failure.
Using perfect form with your elbows planted at your sides, curl the bar up
until it is at your chin. Return to the start position and repeat for 9 more reps.
Rest one minute between sets.
Seated rope curls mid level- 1 set of 12 reps
Attach a single rope handle to the mid pulley on a cable machine. While
seated grab the rope with your left hand and curl the handle straight back
until your arm is fully contracted. There should be no jerking movement, as
all effort should be produced by the biceps muscle. Repeat for a total of 12
reps before switching hands. This exercise is great at maximizing the use of
nearly all fibers in your biceps and causes an intense contraction. Go to
failure on this exercise.
Standing triceps pushdowns- 2 sets of 10 reps
Use either a two-handed rope attachment or a v handle for this exercise.
Fix your elbows at your sides as you press the handle down from chin level
until it reaches full extension in front of your knees. Return the handle to
chest level and press down to full extension again. Repeat for a total of 10
reps. End the first set one rep short of failure and take the second set to
failure. Rest one minute between sets.
Dumbbell triceps kickbacks- 1 set of 12 reps

Use a pair of dumbbells that allow a set of 12 reps to failure. Lean forward while holding the weights at your side with your elbows stationary. Using your lower arms, extend the weights back as far as you can and hold for 2 seconds before returning to the start position. Repeat for 12 reps ending the set at the point of failure.

Routine #2
Dumbbell preacher curls- 2 sets of 10 reps
Use either a standing or seated preacher bench. Press your chest against the bench and place your upper arms on the front of the bench. Lower the weights until you get a good stretch at the bottom. Curl the weights up to the top and squeeze your biceps hard before returning to the beginning position. Repeat for 9 more reps. During this first set stop one rep before hitting failure. Rest 30 seconds then do the second set, ending it at the point of muscular failure.
Dumbbell concentration curls- 1 set of 10 reps
Use a dumbbell that leads to muscular failure at 10 reps
Seated downward cable curls- 1 set of 12 reps
Attach a short two-handed bar or a double strap attachment to the upper pulley on a cable machine. Select a weight that allows you to complete a set of 12 reps, stopping one rep short of failure. Keeping your elbows stationary in front of you at shoulder level, curl the handle down to your shoulders. Pause for one second then return to the start position and repeat for another 11 reps.
Lying triceps extensions omni-contraction- 1 set of 10 reps
Use a pair of dumbbells, a straight bar or an ez-curl bar for this exercise. Use a weight heavy enough to cause failure at the 10-rep mark. Lie down on a flat bench and lower the weight down to either your forehead or just behind your head while keeping your elbows locked in front of you. Press the weight upward in a slight arc motion. Squeeze your triceps muscles hard at the top before beginning the lowering phase. Lower the weight 1/3 of the way and hold for 5 seconds. Lower another 1/3 and hold the weight for 5 seconds. To finish the rep lower the weight almost to the beginning and hold the weight for 5 seconds. Repeat for another 9 reps to failure.
Close grip bench press- 1 set of 12 reps
Use a grip that is about 12 inches apart. Lower the weight to your chest and press it to the top without locking out the bar. Pause for one second then return to the start position. Repeat for a total of 12 reps stopping one rep short of failure.
Seated overhead triceps extensions- 1 set of 12 rep zone partials
Use one dumbbell and grip the weight with both hands at once.
Locking your elbows at the side of your head lower the dumbbell all the way and do 4 reps in the bottom zone. Lift the weight to mid-point and do 4 reps

in the middle zone before doing the final 4 reps in the top third zone. This set should be taken to the point of failure.

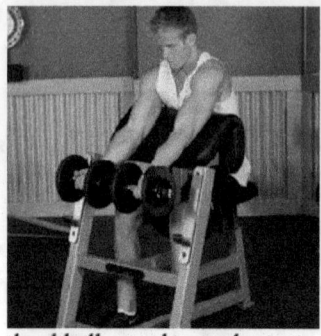 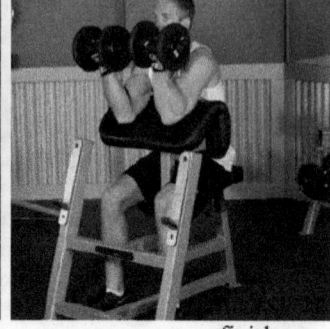

dumbbell preacher curls-start   finish

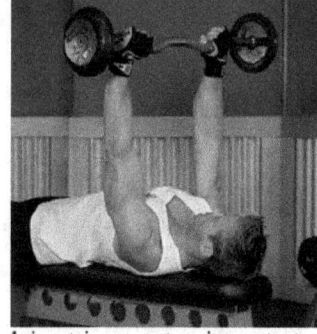 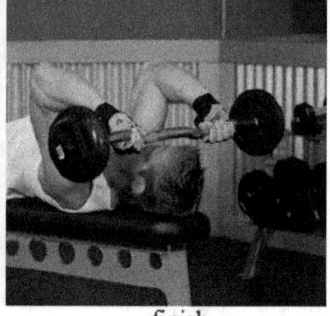

lying triceps extensions-start   finish

Routine #3
Standing dumbbell curls- many sets up and down the rack
Use a moderate weight for your first set and do 12 reps, set the dumbbells down, grab the next heaviest pair and do a second set consisting of 10 reps. Grab the next heaviest and do a set of 8 reps. Continue with this pattern until you hit peak weight for a set of 4 reps then begin decreasing the weight and increasing the reps back up to 6, 8, 10,12 and finally 15 reps, using progressively lighter weights. All sets should be completed to one rep before failure. We are working the biceps muscle with varying weights and rep counts to train all types of muscle fibers and shock the muscles into new growth. This type of training will give you a really great pump as well.
Overhead cable pulldowns- 1 set of 12 holds
Attach a short handle to an overhead pulley attachment and select a weight that allows a maximum hold for 10 seconds.

Pull the handle down ¾ of the way to your chest using a palms-facing grip. hands spaced shoulder width apart. Hold the bar in that position for 10 seconds before returning the weight to the stack for a 10 second rest. Lower the weight slightly then do another 10 second hold. Continue in this fashion for a total of 12. 10 second holds.

The great thing about this routine is after exhausting your biceps with the multiple-set up and down the rack dumbbell curls you change gears and do an advanced HIT variable, static holds, which train your biceps from a different direction using maximum weight loads. This is effective for kick-starting them to new muscle growth. Remember it is very important for you to change your routine often to avoid becoming stale and predictable because your body is very effective at adapting to the stress imposed on it and avoids growing new muscle tissue when it can. This is due to the high energy needed to fuel new muscle growth and maintain it.

Lying inclined dumbbell extensions- 1 set of 12 reps
While lying on an incline bench extend a pair dumbbells overhead using both arms. Begin with the weights just above your head and lift them up using a slightly arcing motion ending with the weights fully extended overhead. This exercise is identical to the lying triceps extensions exercise with a barbell or e-z curl bar. End the set one rep short of muscular failure.
Seated dip machine- 1 set of 12 negative-only reps
Select a weight that is 40% heavier than you typically use in this exercise. Have a partner assist you in pressing the arms of the machine down to the bottom position. After your partner transfers the full load to you resist the force of the weight as the arms press upward. Once the rep is completed have your partner assist with the pressing of the arms down as before. Your assistant should be doing almost all of the work during this phase of the rep. This set should result in complete muscular failure.
Seated triceps extension machine- 1 set of 10 reps
Sit in the machine after selecting a weight that allows the set to be terminated one rep before failure at 10 reps. Fix your elbows on the pad in front of you and grab the handles of the machine. Extend the arms down in front of you until your arms are fully extended. Pause for one second then return to the start position. Repeat for an additional 9 reps.

Shoulders

Routine #1
Seated machine laterals- 1 drop set
Select a weight that allows you to do 12 reps short of failure and complete a set by grabbing the handles and raising the arms of the machine out to the side until they are very slightly above parallel. Pause for one second then

return the arms to the start. Repeat for 11 more reps. Immediately reduce the weight and do another 10 reps short of failure. Reduce the weight again and do 8 reps. Reduce the weight one more time and complete a final 6 reps.

By completing a number of minisets within the one complete set you are working the shoulder muscles numerous times instead of once during a conventional set. This variable leads to a nice pump, which rushes blood and nutrients to the muscle leading to new muscle growth.

Standing dumbbell presses – 1 set of 12 reps
Press two dumbbells overhead while standing. Don't use any momentum or jerking to assist in the lifting of the weight as this will greatly diminish the benefits of this exercise and can lead to shoulder and back injuries. Complete the set with 12 reps short of failure.
Front dumbbell raises- 1 set of 12 reps negative-only
Lift the weights by pressing them and lower them to a count of eight in front of you using a front raise motion. Keep a slight bend in your elbow throughout the exercise. By the 12th negative rep you should be at muscular failure.

Routine #2
Cuban press- 1 set of 12 reps to failure
Stand with your arms at your sides with a dumbbell in each hand. Exhale as you raise the weights by bringing your arms up similar to an upright row movement. When the weights are at shoulder level inhale as you rotate the weights to a shoulder press position. Exhale as you press the weights overhead. Repeat for a total of 12 reps.
Cable rear deltoid raises- 2 sets of 12 reps
Select a weight that allows 12 reps without going to failure. Bend over at the machine and raise the handle in an outward arc until your arm is parallel to the floor. Pause for one second then repeat. Rest one minute then do the second set, taking the set to failure at the 12th rep.

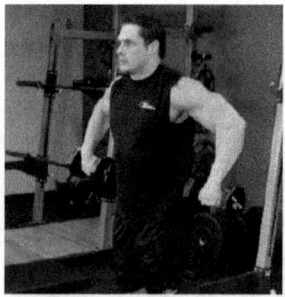
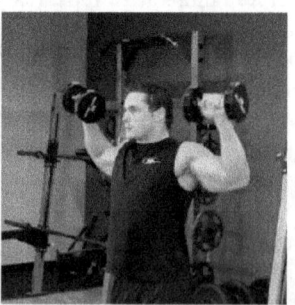

Cuban press-start   mid-point

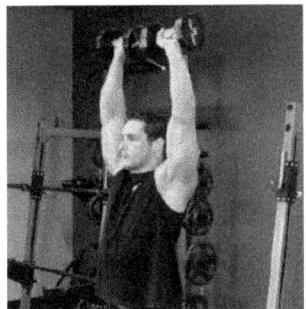
Cuban press- end

Routine #3
Dumbbell rotator cuff rotations- 2 sets of 15 reps
After selecting a pair of light dumbbells, raise them until they are parallel to the floor at shoulder level. Rotate them in a small circular clockwise motion. Gradually increase the size of the circular motion until you are using a 10" diameter circle. Don't go to failure on either of these sets, as we need to be careful not to strain the rotator cuff area. After resting for 30 seconds reduce the weight and do your second set.
Seated machine presses- 1 set of 10 reps
Select a weight that causes failure at 10 reps. Complete the set in the normal fashion.
Lying incline dumbbell extensions- 1 set of 12 reps
Lie flat on your side on an incline bench. Begin by holding the dumbbell against your leg. Raise the dumbbell in an upward arcing motion until it is slightly higher than shoulder level. Repeat for a total of 12 reps.

The workout above is a unique one that you probably will not see in most gyms because the first and last exercises are not well known but are very effective. The first exercise, dumbbell rotator cuff rotations, trains the rotator cuff area using a natural circular motion. This region is often overlooked when training the shoulders. Instead the deltoid muscle is stressed and understandably so because it is responsible for the majority of the shoulder's muscle size. The rotator cuff forms the base for the shoulder's movements so we need to train with this type of exercise on a regular basis.

The second exercise, seated machine presses, is a common movement among trainees. It is a very good power movement and hits all areas of the shoulders pretty equally. Because it is a compound exercise it makes use of the triceps muscles to assist the deltoid muscles in completion of the exercise.

The last exercise, lying incline dumbbell extensions, focuses effort on the middle deltoid area and is very effective because it eliminates bad form and prevents momentum assistance during the exercise.

Abdominals

Routine #1
Stomach crunches- 1 set of 20 crunches to failure
Lie on the floor with your knees pulled in pointing to the ceiling. With your hands behind your head, curl your upper body toward your knees. If properly done you should feel a really intense contraction of your abdominal muscles after a few reps. Tense your abs hard at the top of the movement before returning to the floor. Keep the pressure on the abs and repeat for another 19 reps.
Lying leg raises on bench- 1 set of 20+ reps
Lie on a flat bench with your legs slightly bent. Bring your legs up in an arcing motion until they are ¾ of the way overhead. Lower them to the start position making sure they don't touch at the bottom. Repeat.
Dumbbell side lifts- 1 set of 15 reps per side
Hold a dumbbell in each hand at your sides with your arms straight. Lean to one side and then the other. Continue this back and forth motion until completing all reps.

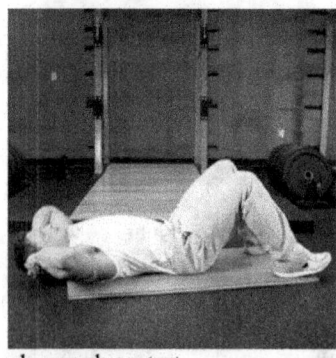 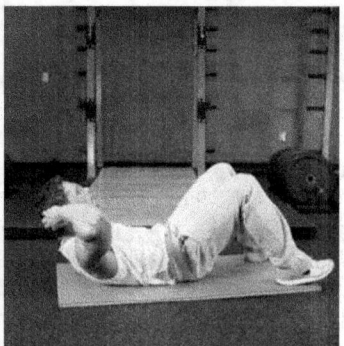

ab crunches-start   finish

Routine #2
Face pulls- 2 sets of 12 reps
Attach a double rope handle to the middle pulley attachment of a cable machine and select a moderate weight. Beginning with straight arms in front of you at face level pull the handle straight into your face. Tense your shoulder muscles hard before returning the handle to the beginning position. Repeat for a total of 12 reps. Rest 30 seconds, reduce the weight and

complete the second set. This exercise focuses on the rear deltoid portion of the muscle. Both sets should be taken until one rep before failure.

Front dumbbell raises- 1 set of 12 reps

Use a weight that causes failure at 12 reps. Stand straight with the dumbbells resting on the front of your legs. Keeping your arms slightly bent, raise the dumbbells in front of you until they are slightly over parallel.

Arnold press- 2 sets of 8 reps

Use two dumbbells for this exercise. Clean the weights to your shoulders using a palms-facing grip. Rotate the weights as you press them overhead until your palms are facing forward. Pause for one second then return to the beginning position. Repeat for another 7 reps. Rest one minute then do the second set in a negative-only fashion. To do this have your partner lift the weights for you and resist the weights as they descend using an 8 count. Continue until you have completed a total of 8 negative reps. You will have to increase the weight from what you used in the first set because you typically can use 40% more weight during a negative rep set.

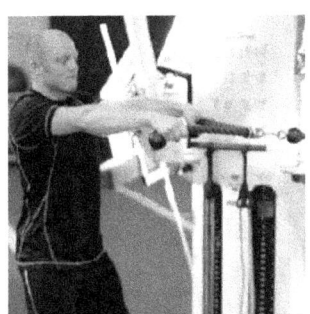 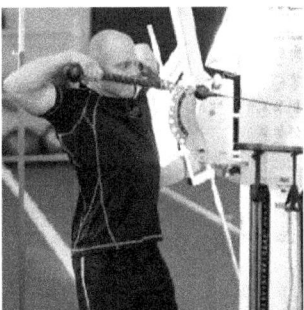

face pulls-start   finish

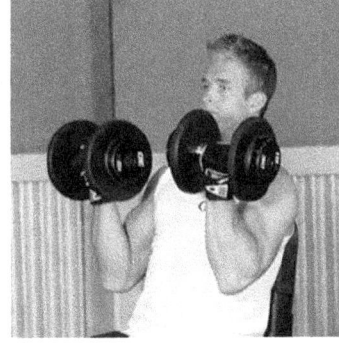 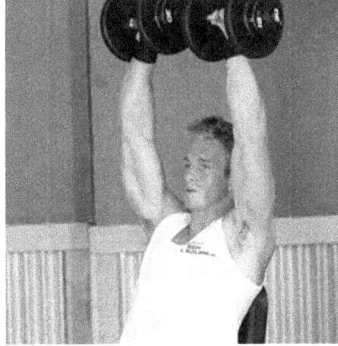

Routine #3
Upright rows- 2 sets of 12 reps

Use either a barbell or a set of dumbbells for this exercise. Using a shoulder width grip lift the weights straight up until they are even with your chin. Pause one second then return the weight to the bottom. Repeat for a total of 12 reps. Rest 30 seconds after reducing the weight and do a second set for 12 reps to failure.

Clean and press- 1 set of 8 reps

Use a set of dumbbells or a barbell with a weight that causes failure at 8 reps in the clean and press. With your grip slightly wider than shoulder width, clean the weight to your shoulders using a rapid motion. Press the weights overhead using a controlled motion but don't lock out the weight at the top. Pause for a second then return the weights to the floor. Repeat for a total of 8 reps.

Side dumbbell laterals- 1 set of 12 reps

Use a pair of dumbbells that allow you to complete 12 reps without going to failure. Standing straight with your arms slightly bent raise the weights from your sides until they are shoulder height. Repeat.

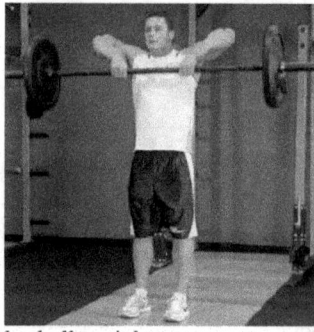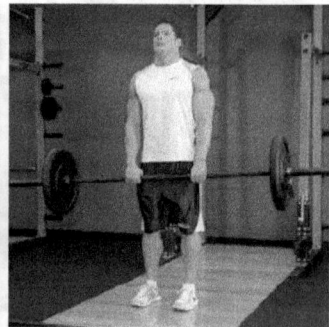

barbell upright row-start   finish

This completes our list of workouts in this section on variable intensity training. While these workouts were specially designed in their order of exercises and sets and reps to maximize your training results to prevent staleness in your training you may substitute exercises from the exercise lists to keep things fresh. Just be sure to substitute an isolation exercise with another isolation exercise in the workout program and a compound exercise with another compound exercise. See the list elsewhere in this manual as well as my high intensity variables book listed at the beginning of this manual.

Traditional High Volume Training

While I am completely convinced that HIT or high intensity training is the best method to generate excellent gains in muscle size and strength, I want to include all of the popular methods of training in this book so I will be outlining the high set traditional type of training, which is most prevalent in bodybuilding training today.

This method goes back to the beginning of muscle training and is the most accepted method of building muscle in use today. It is based on the "if some is good then more is better" approach.

One of the important goals is the attainment of a strong blood engorgement or pump in the muscle. This is the tightness you feel in the muscle after doing a set of moderate to high reps. The thought is that the increased size that you gain temporarily from the pumped muscle translates into permanent muscle size gains. While this hasn't been substantiated in studies it is entirely possible. One thing is for sure, the muscle pump brings much needed muscle building nutrients contained in the blood with it.

The amount of sets used to train each muscle group is typically 10-25 depending on the size and number of different muscles in the group while the number of exercises is 3-6.

Because of the amount of different exercises used per group a trainee is able to hit a muscle from multiple angles, which affects it in a new and different way. This often will stimulate new growth. So while I advocate the HIT, or scientific approach to bodybuilding and fitness training, there are some advantages to the HV, or high volume approach.

The amount of rest between sets and rep counts differ depending on the goal(s) of the training. If the goal is to bulk up then heavier weights and lower rep counts are used, generally in the 3-6 range with 1-2 minutes rest between sets. If cutting up, or losing fat is the goal then the rep count changes to 10-15 with up to 30 seconds rest between sets. One thing to keep in mind though is the fact that to decrease fat you should attempt to increase your muscle mass. Since muscle burns far more calories than other tissue it will assist greatly in fat loss by calorie burning. This is best accomplished with a moderate rep count in the 8-12 range.

While sets are sometimes taken to muscular failure, generally the sets are terminated one to two reps short of failure. This is necessary because it is impossible to generate maximum intensity when training with higher sets because it becomes necessary to pace oneself in order to complete the desired amount of sets. The goal is to complete a specific amount of sets instead of attaining a high level of intensity.

You will hear that a bodybuilder has increased his intensity level by increasing the amount of sets that he/she is using in their training. This is impossible for the reason mentioned above. Remember from the HIT portion of this manual, If intensity increases the amount of work (sets) needs to decrease and vice versa.

HV-High Volume Training Routines

Legs

Routine#1
Leg extensions- 4 sets of 15 reps
Do one set of 15 reps, stopping the set one rep before failure. Rest one minute then do the next set in the same fashion. Complete the final sets in the same way.
Barbell squats- 4 sets of 8,10,15,20 reps
Do the first set of 8 reps, rest one minute then do a second set of 10 reps. Complete the final sets in the same way.
Dumbbell lunges- 3 sets of 12 reps per leg
Hold a dumbbell in each hand; arms should be fully extended by your sides. Step forward by taking a deep, long step. Push off with your forward leg until you are standing erect. Repeat with your other leg. Continue until you have completed 12 reps per leg.
Leg curls- 3 sets of 15 reps
Use a standing, lying or seated leg curl machine for this one. Select a weight that allows you to complete 15 controlled reps without going to failure and curl the weight until your foot almost touches your buttocks. Repeat for a total of 15 reps.
Calf raises- 3 sets of 15 reps
Use a machine if you have one available. Select a heavy weight and do 15 reps, rest one minute then do the second set. Complete the final set after a one minute rest.

Routine#2
Leg press- 4 sets of 4,8,12,15 reps
Use a leg press machine with a selectorized stack using horizontal positioning or one that plate loads where you lie under it if a selectorized one isn't available. Place your feet on the plate slightly wider than shoulder width. Press the plate all the way but don't lockout. Hold for one second then return to the start position. Complete 4 reps this set, rest then progress through the final sets in the same way, resting one minute between sets.
Dumbbell squats-4 sets of 8,12,15,20 reps

This exercise eliminates the need for squat racks and a spotter because you hold one or two dumbbells in a position where you could safely drop it if you get stuck.

Hold a dumbbell in front of you at chest level with both hands. Alternatively, you can hold two dumbbells, one in each hand, at your sides. Use a stance that is slightly wider than shoulder width and keep your head up by looking straight ahead throughout the exercise. Descend as far as you can comfortably, preferably all the way down as that trains your hamstring muscles in addition to your quadriceps, or front thigh muscles. Breathe deeply and press yourself up to the top. Repeat for 8 reps. Rest 1-1.5 minutes and do the next set. Continue until you have completed all sets.

Leg extensions- 3 sets of 15 reps

Complete three sets of leg extensions with a minute of rest between them. On each rep extend the machine arms to the top and flex your thighs hard to increase the contraction in your muscles.

Seated calf raises 3 sets of 15 reps

Select a weight that comes close to failure at 15 reps. Get a full stretch by placing the ball of your feet on the foot block and letting the weight press your heel toward the floor. Lift your heels up as far as you can to get a full contraction. Flex your calves hard at the top before returning to the start position. Repeat, resting one minute between sets.

Routine#3

Leg presses-supersetted with

Leg extensions- 3 supersets

Do a set of 15 leg presses. As soon as you complete the set perform a set of 15 leg extensions. Rest one minute then repeat the superset. Do a third superset cycle in the same way.

Leg lunges- 3 sets of 12 lunges per leg

Use one dumbbell in each hand, holding them at your sides. Take a long step forward and bend down low before pushing back with your extended leg. Repeat with the other leg. Continue alternating legs until you have completed 12 lunges with each leg.

Stiff legged deadlifts- 3 sets of 10, 12, 15 reps

Stand with legs locked and bend down and grab a barbell or two dumbbells. Keeping your legs straight stand up with the bar and extend yourself backward as in a regular deadlift. Rest one minute between sets before doing the next set. This exercise effectively works the hamstring muscles on the back of your upper legs.

Donkey calf raises- 3 sets of 12 reps

Bend over until you are horizontal and place your arms on the bench. Have a partner sit on your back to add weight. Get a good stretch by letting the weight push the heels of your feet toward the floor. Press your heels up and flex your calves to get a strong contraction. Repeat the final sets with a one minute rest between them.

Back

Routine#1
Pullovers- 3 sets of 10 reps
If no pullover machine is available use a dumbbell and bench. Lay against the bench with your back facing the bench. Inhale deeply as you extend the dumbbell behind you down over the bench. Exhale as you bring the dumbbell back over your head. Repeat for a total of 10 reps, resting one minute between sets. This exercise is an isolation exercise, which means most of the effort is generated by the back muscles. We will follow it with a compound exercise, which uses fresh muscles to assist the back in completion of the exercise. This allows us to train the back muscles harder giving us better results.
Barbell rows- 3 sets of 10 reps
Immediately after finishing pullovers bend over a pre-loaded barbell and grip the bar slightly wider than shoulder width. Pull the bar to your lower chest and squeeze your back muscles hard. Repeat for a total of 10 reps. Rest one minute then do the next set. Complete the final set the same way.
Cable pulldowns- 3 sets of 12 reps
Use a single cable handle, which allows you to train one side of your back at a time. As you pull the handle to your chest turn the handle in a circle to change your grip. This hits your back from different angles, which changes the exercise slightly. Lean back slightly and extend your arms up to get a full stretch.
Lower back extensions- 3 sets of 12 reps
Select a moderately heavy weight. Carefully press against the machine arm to push yourself backward until fully extended. Pause for one second then repeat.

Routine#2
One arm dumbbell rows- 3 sets of 8, 12, 15 reps
Brace one hand against the dumbbell rack while you row a dumbbell with the other hand. At the beginning of the exercise let the weight pull your arm down for a full stretch. Row the weight until it touches your chest. Repeat for 8 reps for the first set, 12 reps for the second and 15 for the final set.
Pull-ups- 2 sets of 10 reps
Starting from a stretched position pull yourself up to do a "pull-up". Repeat for a total of 10 reps. Rest one to two minutes between sets.
If you can complete 10 reps easily add weight via a dip belt.
Straight arm pulldowns- 3 sets of 10 reps

Stand in front of a cable machine after attaching a straight bar to the high pulley attachment. Keep your arms locked straight and pull the bar down until the bar is at your thighs. Squeeze your lats hard to get an intense contraction before returning to the top position. Repeat for a total of 10 reps. Rest one minute between sets.

Inclined barbell rows- 4 sets of 8, 10, 12, reps

Load a barbell with a moderate weight and place it under an inclined bench. Grab the bar with a medium grip after lying face down on the bench and pull it up until it touches the bench. Tense your back muscles hard and return the bar to the floor. Rest 1.5 minutes between sets. Adjust the weight on the bar so you are able to complete the appropriate rep count in each set.

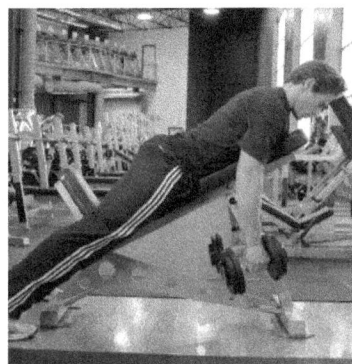 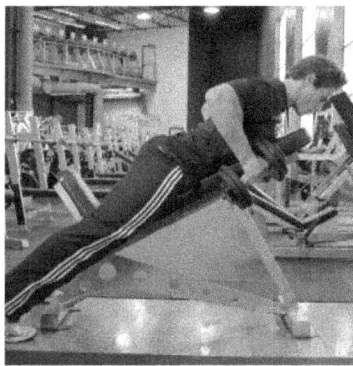

incline dumbbell row-start   finish

Routine#3

Pullovers on machine- 1 set of 12 reps

Trisetted

One arm dumbbell rows- 1 set of 8 reps

Trisetted

Middle back shrug- 1 sets of 12 reps

Lie face down on an incline bench after selecting two heavy dumbbells. Keeping your arms straight shrug the weights up as far as you can and squeeze your shoulder and back muscles as hard as you can before repeating.

This exercise is not as common as some other back exercises but is very effective at building up the upper back muscle area as well as the trap region. Heavy weights can be used in this exercise but don't overdue it or you will begin to compensate by using other muscles to assist in the lifting of the weight. You can use a flat or incline bench, as they are both equally effective and hit the muscles from different angles.

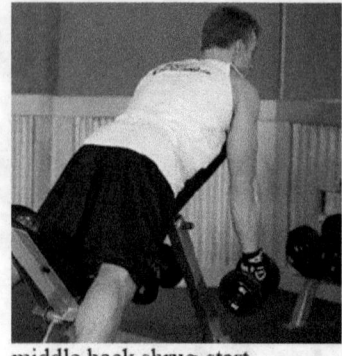 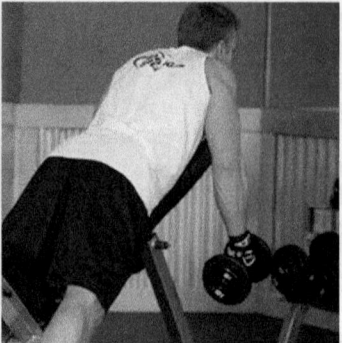

middle back shrug-start   finish

After doing one cycle of these exercises rest 1.5 minutes before repeating the series of three exercises. Perform two cycles as a beginner and progress to 3-4 cycles as you become more advanced.

Chest

Routine#1
Dumbbell flyes- 1 set of 8 reps
Trisetted
Barbell bench press- 1 set of 8 reps
Trisetted
Cable crossovers mid-pulley- 1 set of 12 reps
Attach a handle to the mid pulley on a cable machine after selecting a moderate weight. Stand with your back facing the machine. Keeping your arms slightly bent pull the handle across your chest in a downward arcing motion. Squeeze your pec muscles hard before repeating the movement.

Do one triset cycle then rest for 90 seconds before repeating the cycle. As a beginner do two cycles and progress up to 3-4 cycles as a more advanced trainee.

Routine#2
Machine inclined bench press- many sets of 8, 10, 12 reps per set
Select a weight that allows 8 reps for the first set. Complete that set before changing the weight for a 10 reps set. For the next set do a total of 12 reps. Keep changing the weight and completing sets of 8, 10 and 12 reps by reducing the resistance as your muscles become more exhausted with your efforts. Total sets should be in the range of 8-12 as experience dictates. Rest one minute between sets at most.

64

Routine#3

Decline bench press- 3 sets of 8, 10, 12 reps

Use a decline bench press machine if one is available. If not, a good decline or adjustable bench will work fine. Use either a barbell or a pair of dumbbells with a moderate weight. Lower the weight to a point below your nipples, pause for one second then press up in a smooth motion. Do not lock out. After completing 8 reps rest for one minute then do the second set of 10 reps. Your last set will consist of 12 reps.

Dumbbell flyes- 3 sets of 8, 10, 12 reps

Use a pair of dumbbells and complete a set of 8 reps while lying on a flat bench. Get a good stretch at the bottom by bringing the dumbbells as far down as is comfortable before lifting them in an arcing motion. Don't let the weights touch at the top as that removes the tension from your muscles, which is something we want to avoid. Rest one minute between sets.

Machine dips-2 sets of 10 reps + 3 negative reps

Lean forward in the dip machine to concentrate the exercise to your chest. Press the machine arms down to the point before lockout, hold for one second then return to the top. Complete 10 reps in the first set. After resting for one minute do the second set of 10 reps followed by 3 negative-only reps. To do these have a partner push the machine arms to the bottom position then transfer the resistance to you. Resist the weight as it returns to the stack to a count of 8.

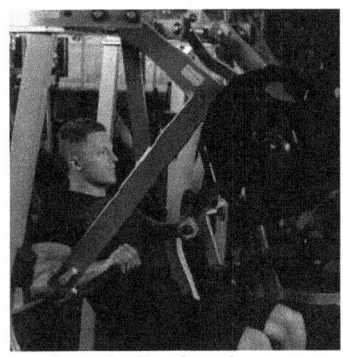 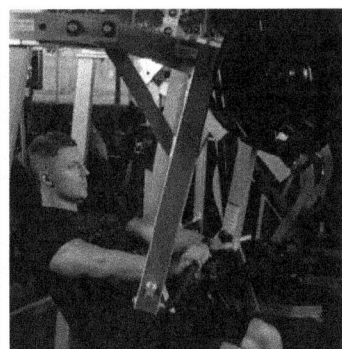

machine decline bench press-start   finish

Muscle fiber makeup

The reason we have been using multiple sets with different rep schemes in this section is the first rep count, 8, works mostly the fast twitch fibers, 10 reps train mixed fast twitch/slow twitch and 12 reps train slow twitch. This allows us to concentrate our efforts on training the entire muscle which leads to maximum muscle growth.

Each individual has a different fiber composition. Some have more fast twitch- some have more slow twitch and some have a more mixed fiber makeup. The fast twitch fibers are responsible for most muscle size in an individual. The bodybuilders with the most muscle size and favorable genetics for muscle bulk have the most fast twitch fibers in a given muscle.

Keep in mind, however, that different muscles in the same person have completely different fiber types so a bodybuilder will have excellent development in one muscle group while he is lacking in another muscle group. Therefore, it is very important to learn each of your muscle groups' fiber makeup so you can individualize your workouts to achieve maximum results.

Shoulders

Routine#1
Seated dumbbell side lateral raises- 1 set of 12 reps
Sit on a flat bench straddling it. Keep your arms slightly bent and lift the weights until they reach shoulder height out to your side. Pause one second then lower them back down, repeating for a total of 12 reps. This exercise trains the entire shoulder but concentrates on the middle head of the deltoid.
Seated front lateral raises- 1 set of 12 reps
Sit on a flat bench straddling it as noted above. Lift the dumbbells straight up in front of you keeping your arms slightly bent until they reach shoulder height. Pause for one second then lower, completing a total of 12 reps.
Cable internal rotation- 2 sets of 15 reps
Sit next to a low pulley sideways (with legs stretched in front of you or crossed) and grasp the single hand cable attachment with the arm nearest to the cable. If one is available use a flat bench to sit on instead.
Position your elbow against your side with it bent at 90 degrees and pointing towards the pulley. This will be your starting position.
Pull the single hand cable attachment toward your body by internally rotating your shoulder until your forearm is across your abs. Your forearm should be perpendicular to your torso at all times. Lower steadily back to the initial position. Repeat for a total of 15 reps and switch arms.
Dumbbell presses- 4 sets of 6, 8, 10, 12 reps
Do your first set of 6 reps with a fairly heavy weight that taxes your muscles almost to failure. After resting one minute do the second set of 8 reps with a weight that is slightly lighter than the first set. Rest one minute then complete the final two sets in the same manner.

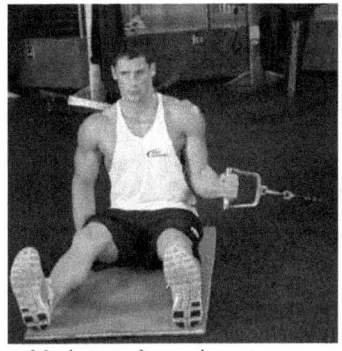 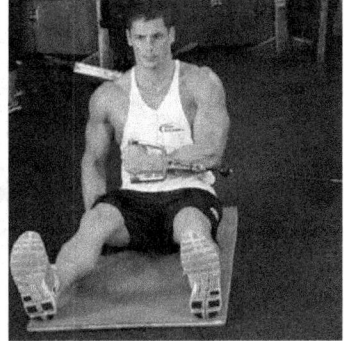

cable internal rotation-start   finish

Routine#2

Machine press behind neck- 3 sets of 6, 8, 10 reps
Select a moderately heavy weight for the first set of 6 reps. Sit with your back facing the press machine. Grab the handles and press them up to just before the lockout position. Pause for one second then return to the beginning position. Repeat for a total of 6 reps, rest then perform the next set of 8 reps the same way. Complete the final two sets the same way.

Band angle press- 3 sets of 10 reps
This is an exercise that I designed to be effective at stimulating growth in the shoulder muscle in a unique way. Attach two strength bands to the bottom on a bench. Face away from the bands, and while holding them, press them up at an angle in front of you. The movement should resemble an upright incline bench press with a steeper angle upwards to put the effort on the shoulders instead of the chest. At the top, which is the point of maximum contraction, tense your deltoids hard to stimulate the muscles to contract even harder. Return to the bottom and repeat for a total of 10 reps. Rest one minute between sets and reduce the band resistance as necessary to allow completion of 10 reps.

Machine shrugs- 4 sets of 6, 8, 10, 12 reps
If an older Nautilus Shrug machine is available use that for this exercise as that machine is fantastic at isolating the traps and working them hard.
If you don't have access to that machine use a barbell or a pair of heavy dumbbells. Stand, holding the weights with straight arms. Exhale as you shrug your shoulders as far up as you can and hold for three seconds before lowering the weights. For your first set do 6 reps, rest one minute then complete the second set. Complete the last sets in the same way.

Very heavy weights can be used in this exercise, so really load the machine or barbell up with lots of weight to thicken the trap muscles.

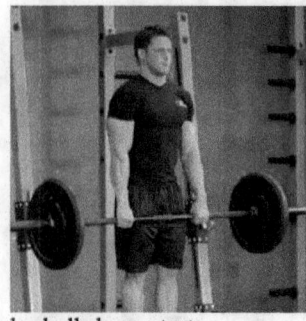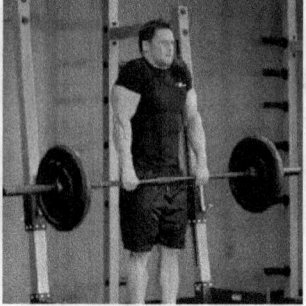

barbell shrug-start   finish

Routine#3

Lying incline reverse lateral raises- 2 sets of 10 reps

Lie face down on an incline bench. Keeping your arms slightly bent lift two dumbbells upward in a backward arcing motion until they are parallel with the floor. Complete a total of 10 reps, rest one minute and then finish the second set of 10 reps. As a variation, do these while lying on a flat bench.

Presses in a power rack- 4 sets of 6, 8, 10, 12 reps

Place the pins in the rack so the barbell is located at the mid-point of a barbell press. After loading the bar with a heavier than usual weight, press it up until just before lockout then lower slowly to a count of 5. Repeat for a total of 6 reps. Move the pins to the ¾ point in the press and do some short presses until just prior to lockout. After finishing that set move the pins to the beginning position of the press and do 10 full reps with a moderate weight. Reduce the weight and complete 12 reps.

Kettlebell round the worlds- 2 sets of 12 reps

Grab a moderately heavy kettlebell with both hands. Stand erect and pass the kettlebell through your legs and circle around your body in a figure '8'. Complete 12 reps then reverse the figure '8' motion and finish with 12 reps in that direction. This movement works your rotator cuffs as well as the entire shoulder structure.

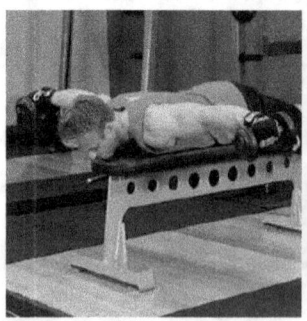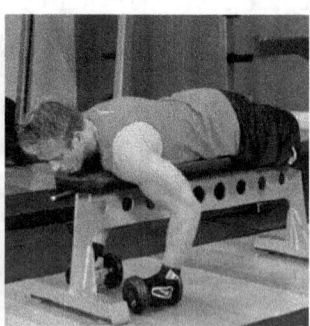

lying rear delt raise-start   finish

Arms

Routine#1
Barbell curls 21's- 2 sets of 10 reps
Load the bar with a moderate weight. Curl the bar up $1/3^{rd}$ of the way.
Return to the bottom and curl the bar to the midpoint and return. Curl the bar
using a full rep. This counts as one rep. Repeat for a total of 10 of these reps.
This exercise changes the barbell curl into a new exercise because of the
multiple contractions per rep (3) that are completed. The typical set has one
contraction per rep.
Concentration curl- 2 sets of 8 reps per arm
Use a moderate dumbbell for this exercise. Lean over and place the elbow of
the arm you're training on your knee on the same side. Curl the weight up to
your chin and return. Repeat for a total of 8 reps before changing arms.
Palms-facing pulldowns- 3 sets of 8, 10, 12 reps
Attach a medium width curved handle to an overhead pulley on a cable
machine. Using a palms-facing grip that is slightly narrower than shoulder
width pull the bar down to your upper chest. Repeat for 8 reps on the first
set. After reducing the weight slightly do a second set of 10 reps. Finish by
completing a final set of 12 reps. All sets have a 60 second rest period
between them.
Seated dumbbell triceps extensions-supersetted
Sit on a bench while holding one dumbbell with two hands behind your
head. Keep your elbows in a fixed position on the side of your head and
press the weight up. Repeat.
Triceps kickbacks- supersetted
Lean forward and brace yourself while holding a dumbbell in each hand.
Keep your elbows planted at your sides and extend them as far back as you
can. Repeat.
Seated dips- supersetted
Sit upright in a dip machine after selecting a moderate weight on the stack.
Press the arms of the machine all the way to the bottom and return. Keep
your upper arms by your side throughout. Repeat.
Do a total of 3 supersets of each of these exercises with no rest between
them. The first superset will be 8 reps in each exercise, 10 in the second and
10 in the final superset.
Reverse wrist curls- 2 sets of 15 reps
Grip a barbell with an overhand grip. Extend your hands upward as far as
you can. Repeat.
Wrist rollers- 1 set of 6 windups
Attach a weight plate to a wrist roller. Curl the rope onto the handle using a
palms-up grip. Let the weight drop back to the floor and repeat for a total of
6 wind-ups.

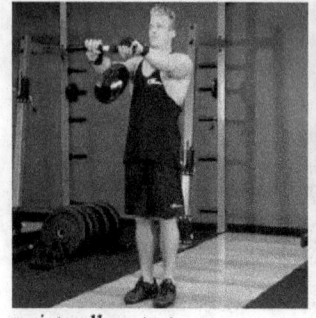 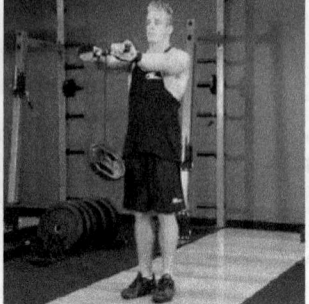

wrist roller-start   finish

Routine#2

Bench dumbbell curls- 3 sets of 8, 10, 12 reps
Lie flat face down on an incline bench. Curl two dumbbells up as far as you can and return. Do a total of 8 reps on the first set, 10 on the second and 12 on the final set.

Machine curls- 3 sets of 6, 8, 10 reps
Select a moderate weight, place your elbows on the pads of the machine and curl the handles up to your chin and return. Repeat for a total of 6 reps on the first set, 8 on the second and 10 during the final set. Rest 30 seconds between sets.

Rope curls high pulley- 2 sets of 10 reps
Attach a single rope handle to the high pulley on a cable machine. Set your elbow in front of you and maintain that position throughout the exercise. Curl the rope all the way to the back of your head and flex your bicep muscle hard. Do 10 reps with your left arm before switching to your right. Rest one minute between sets.

Lying triceps extensions (skull crushers)- 2 sets of 8 reps
Use an ez-curl bar or two dumbbells for this exercise. Lie on a flat bench face up. Lower the weight to your forehead until it almost touches. Make sure your elbows are kept in a fixed position in front of you. Press the weight out all the way. Repeat for 8 reps. Rest one minute then complete the second set.

Close-grip bench presses- 4 sets of 6, 8, 10, 12 reps
Lie on a flat bench. Lower a moderately weighted barbell using an 18" grip down to your chest and press to lockout. Repeat for 6 reps the first set, 8 the second, 10 the third and 12 during the final set. Rest one minute between sets.

Seated machine triceps extensions- 2 sets of 8 and 10 reps
Sit in a triceps extension machine and select a moderate weight. Place your elbows on the pad in front of you and grab the handles of the machine. Press the arms out all the way and flex your triceps hard. Return the arms to the

beginning and repeat for a total of 8 reps. Rest one minute then complete a set of 10 reps.

Reverse curls- 2 sets of 12 reps

Use a standard barbell with less weight than you normally use in a barbell curl. Grab the bar with an overhand grip and curl it up all the way. Return to the start position and repeat for a total of 12 reps. Complete a second set after resting for one minute.

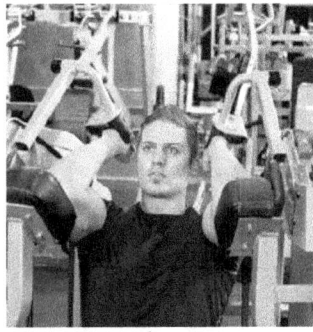 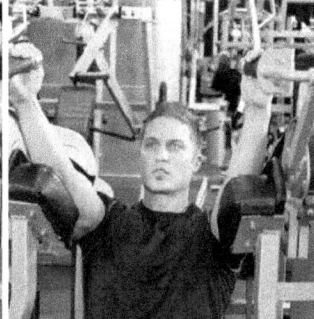

triceps extensions-start   finish

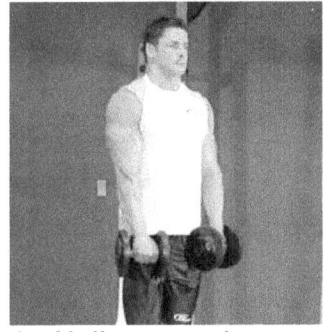 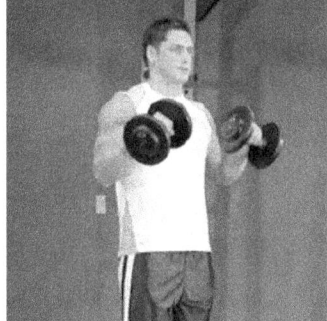

dumbbell reverse curl-start   finish

Routine#3

Triceps cable pressdowns-4 sets of 6, 8, 10, 12 reps

Stand straight and anchor your elbows at your side. Press a triceps handle or rope down in front of you to full extension and return. Complete 6 reps in the first set, rest a minute then continue.

Overhead dumbbell triceps extensions- 3 sets of 10 reps

Sit on a flat bench and anchor your elbows at the side of your head. Lift the weights until they are fully extended overhead. Flex your triceps hard at the top to increase the power of the contraction before returning to the bottom. Complete 10 reps, rest one minute then continue.

Standing bar dips- 2 sets of 8 negative reps

Use a weight belt to add resistance if needed. Step up to full extension using your legs. Stand erect to concentrate the effort on your Triceps. If you lean forward it places the effort on your chest, which isn't what we are looking for. Lower yourself to a count of 8 then repeat. Continue until you complete 8 reps. Rest one minute then complete the final set.

Lying cable curls- 2 sets of 10 reps

Attach a double rope handle to an overhead pulley on a cable machine. Lie flat on the bench in front of the machine. Pull the handle down in a curling motion until it is at your face. Tense your biceps muscles hard and return. Complete a total of 10 reps, rest one minute then finish the final set of 10.

Standing band curls- 2 sets of 8, 10 reps

Stand on a moderate resistance band with both feet. Using both arms curl the band up to complete a full curl. Instead of returning to the bottom position right away, lower one third of the way and do a series of pulsating reps. These are done by doing short, quick curling motions up and down in this zone to cause a strong contraction in the muscle. After doing a series of these, lower down to the mid-point zone and do a series of pulsating reps in that zone. Finally, lower to the beginning position and finish the rep with a series of pulsating reps there. Complete two sets with a one-minute rest period in between.

Barbell rows with palms facing front- 2 sets of 8 reps

Do a standard set of barbell rows with the exception of gripping the bar with your palms facing front on the bar. This shifts the focus of the exercise to the biceps muscles from the back muscles. This is a compound exercise, which uses your fresh back muscles to work your biceps past the point of failure. Both the sets in this exercise should be to failure with a one-minute rest period in between. Reduce the weight on the bar after the initial set as needed.

Heavy-duty grip squeezes- 2 sets with each hand

Use a good pair of grippers for this exercise.

Squeeze the grippers for 15-20 reps each hand. After resting one minute squeeze them again except this time hold the gripper closed for one second on each rep before doing the next rep. This adds additional crushing strength training to this exercise.

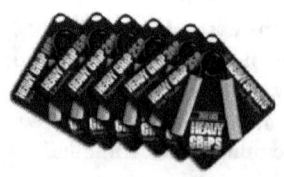

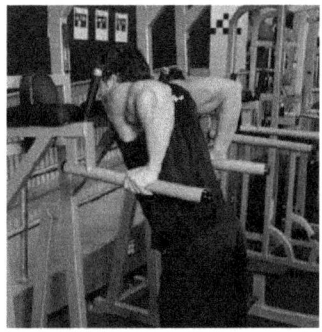
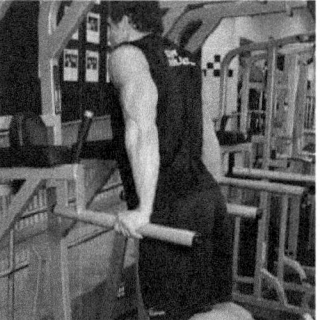

bar dips-start   finish

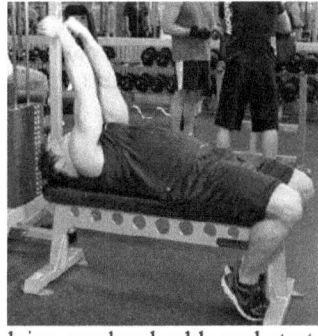
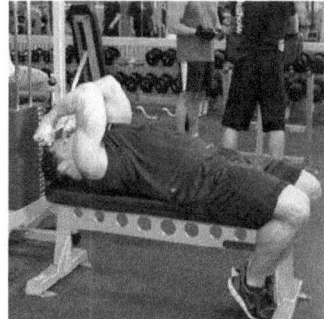

lying overhead cable curl-start   finish

I have outlined some techniques, which can be used with the high volume
approach. The set counts I have used in this section are pretty conservative
compared with other high volume routines but keep in mind when
comparing them to the training programs you see in the bodybuilding
magazines, the routines in the magazines are designed for competitive
bodybuilders who are using chemically enhanced training. In other
words…anabolic steroids and human growth hormone as well as other
drugs. This is something I am very strongly opposed to as it leads to poor
health and often death. In my opinion, and hopefully yours, it isn't worth
risking your health to attain a better physique or bodybuilding title. Instead
we need to be concerned with building our overall health. Larger, stronger
muscles are a part of that.

Supplements to help you grow

There are supplements, however, that help boost your ability to grow larger
muscles. Many of these work by boosting your testosterone and human
growth hormone. Some work by giving you more energy to train intensely

73

while others boost the protein available for your muscles to repair and grow larger after training. We'll explore some of the ones I recommend here.

Recuperative agents

Creatine
This substance is a metabolite of an amino acid. Creatine is available in pill form but is mostly taken in powder form. It has been scientifically proven to aid in muscle strength and size increase in weight trainees. This is largely due to its ability to pull water into the muscles, which increases protein synthesis. This is the process by which the body increases the size of a muscle. Creatine also increases ATP stores which causes the body to produce more energy and power for short periods, such as with weight training, sprinting, football and the like. It has not been shown to be effective at increasing endurance so its usefulness for long distance running is very limited.

But for our concern-the building of new muscle tissue and the production of additional strength- it is the perfect nutritional supplement. As far as safety goes, because creatine is one of the most studied supplements, and it has been found to be completely safe, we can comfortably use it to help us with our training goals. In fact, there are many medical studies underway to further explore health benefits that have been discovered with creatine use.

I recommend you use creatine powder not liquids because the liquids tend to be less stable than regular creatine powder and break down in your blood stream. Use creatine monohydrate, not one of the fancy creatine esters or the like. Make sure you purchase a good brand to avoid the use of an inferior, low-grade product. Adding fruit juice triggers the release of insulin, which drives more of the creatine into the muscle. Be careful as to dosage. Most manufacturers recommend an initial loading phase, which is designed to saturate your muscles with creatine. After that you switch to a maintenance phase for the duration.

L-Glutamine
This is an abundant amino acid found mostly in skeletal muscle tissue in the body. It is an important building block for the body's immune system and is involved in protein synthesis. It has been shown to be an effective recuperative agent after engaging in high intensity activity such as weight training. Buy a good brand and follow the dosage instructions on the package.

Protein

Protein is the building block of muscle and thus is a very important supplement if you want to maintain and build new muscle. Whey protein is the favorite protein powder of bodybuilders and for good reason, it is absorbed fast into the bloodstream and is of good quality. It is made from by-products of the cheese-making industry, whey. Most of the protein powders you encounter on the market will consist of whey protein.

Another good quality protein is casein. Also of dairy origin, it is extracted from milk and is a slower digested protein, making it an ideal complement to whey which is rapidly absorbed and dissipates more readily.

Egg protein is a very good quality protein and can be obtained from eggs and protein powders made from eggs. It is digested slower and stays in your system longer.

Soy protein is a plant-based protein, and while a fairly good protein, is considered to be inferior to the others. In fact, soy products in general have been shown to raise the female hormone estrogen levels in the body. Something male bodybuilders, and men in general, do not want.

I recommend a good quality whey protein mixed with either casein or egg protein to balance out the protein life cycle in your bloodstream.

Pre-workout drinks

These drinks can be a great way to build up energy prior to a workout and help increase your pump during a training session. They are a bit controversial due to their ingredient list. Some experts feel that their use could be dangerous, especially if they are used extensively. They have several ingredients that are strong stimulants such as caffeine as well as other ingredients such as beta alanine, and alpha keto-glutarate. Both of these last two ingredients are vasodilators, which dilate, or open up your blood vessels, which really pumps up your muscles. While this is a plus, remember that excessive caffeine can overload your heart and skyrocket your blood pressure. If you use these products take a conservative dosage and you should reap the benefits without any negative side effects but make sure you are heart-healthy first.

Testosterone Boosters

There are several herbal supplements that have been researched and found to be effective at stimulating your body to produce additional testosterone. Fenugreek has been shown to raise test levels an average of 5.5-6 percent over a short period. While this isn't significant, it certainly is a boost in testosterone. Boron is another supplement that has been shown to increase free testosterone. It seems to do this by reducing the testosterone-binding protein globulin in the bloodstream, causing an increase in free testosterone of 28%. This is a substantial increase, and while it won't give you dramatic gains, causes a potential cumulative positive effect. What's more, it has been shown to decrease men's chances of contracting prostate cancer. Tongkat Ali has been shown in animal studies to increase total testosterone by 30% safely. This is an herbal medicine that has been used in the Far East for centuries to treat low testosterone levels.

Ginger has been shown in animal studies to raise testosterone levels but at this time it isn't known to what level.

Give some of these a try and see what results you can produce with a combination of hard training and supplementation.

Aromatase Inhibitors

Your body converts some of the testosterone in your body to the female hormone estrogen using Aromatase, an enzyme found in the liver responsible for converting male hormone to female hormone.

While it is necessary to have both testosterone (male) and estrogen (female) hormones, it becomes a problem for the male bodybuilder when too much of the male hormone is converted to the female one.

As a man's testosterone rises due to natural causes or steroids, more is converted to estrogen, causing female breast characteristics and fat gain among other side effects. One way to prevent this is to use either drug or natural Aromatase inhibitors. It is desirable to use natural Aromatase inhibitors due to the side effects that the drug versions can produce.

Some natural Aromatase inhibitors are Chrysin, Myomin and Diindoylymethane or DIM, a substance common in broccoli, kale and cauliflower. Chrysin is a flavone that has proven to be a very effective Aromatase inhibitor as is Myomin. The best way to maximize benefits of these nutraceuticals is to buy a product that contains several of these compounds from a reputable company and take the recommended dosage.

One of the effects of these medications/supplements is an increase in testosterone, the male hormone most responsible for increasing protein synthesis and muscle mass in the body. As you prevent conversion of testosterone to estrogen, your glands continue to produce additional testosterone leading to a higher level than before taking the Aromatase-inhibiting supplements.

Beta Alanine

This is a non-essential amino acid that is produced in the liver. It is also obtained in the diet from meat and poultry. It combines with the amino acid Histidine to form the dipeptide Carnosine, which is what gives the benefits from Beta Alanine supplementation. Carnosine works by increasing your muscle's ability to buffer hydrogen ions, which are produced when lactate levels rise during intense exercise such as weight training. This increases the muscle's ability to maintain stronger contractions for longer periods of time during exercise. It does this by lowering the lactic acid buildup thereby extending one's ability to maintain strength during a workout. Take between 3-6 grams per day for full benefits.

BCAA'S

The branched-chain amino acids, or BCAAs, are the three essential amino acids leucine, isoleucine, and valine. In addition to increasing muscle growth, the amino acid leucine stimulates muscle protein synthesis and increases the hormone insulin in the bloodstream. As well as the regulation of sugar in the blood, insulin is anabolic, meaning that it stimulates additional protein synthesis. These aminos also increase human growth hormone in the body, which is a very important hormone when it comes to building muscle and burning fat.

Advanced Workouts

Special Ultra-High Intensity Routines

This specialty training includes the use of advanced HIT variables such as forces reps, negatives, static holds, rolling static partials, partials, isometric holds, Infitonic, strip sets and more. While we used these principles in the first section on high intensity training, we typically used a to-failure set on one exercise and a HIT variable on another set or two while training a particular muscle group. In this phase we are going to lower our set count keeping with the formula-the higher the intensity the lower the volume of work. This helps us to use just the proper amount of training (workload) to stimulate muscle gains and no more. The use of more training than is necessary to stimulate maximum growth is a negative and can lead to overtraining.

To accomplish ratcheting up of intensity we will use 2-3 different HIT variables in one set of an exercise enabling us to achieve maximum results from one total set for smaller muscle groups and two total sets for larger muscle groups.

Machines are the best pieces of equipment to use with this type of training as they place the muscles in the proper groove and have cams that have been specially engineered to give maximum stimulation to the muscle(s) being trained. They are safer to use and are much easier to change the weight quickly. This being said, free weights such as dumbbells and barbells are effective with this training.

The goal of this training is to place the maximum amount of stress safely on the muscle in the shortest period of time-maximizing growth stimulation in the least amount of time. Workouts typically last only 15-20 minutes with this method.

Legs

Routine#1
Leg extensions- 1 set of 12 reps + negatives+static holds
Select a weight that causes failure at 12 reps. After hitting failure have your partner lift the arms of the machine to the full extension position then transfer the resistance to your legs. Lower slowly to a count of 8. Repeat until you lose control of the downward motion. Have your partner lift the arms of the machine into the full extension position. Hold the weight in this position for a 10 count then lower. Reduce the weight then repeat for another 10-second hold. Continue for three more holds then move immediately to the leg press machine.
Leg presses- 1 set of 12 reps+negative-accentuated reps+ rolling static partials
Complete 12 reps to failure. After completing those press the footplate to the top and resist the weight with your left leg only as it descends. Press the plate up to the top again and resist the weight with your right leg in the same way. Continue until unable to safely control the downward descent of the weight.

Reduce the weight then press the weight up and do a series of short, six-inch pulsing type reps and do a hold in the middle of one of the reps. Continue by doing additional short pulsing reps with holds in various parts of the reps. The holds should be for a duration of 5 seconds each. After completion of these two sets your legs should be extremely tired.
Calf raises- 1 set of 12 reps+ rolling static partials

Routine#2
Barbell squats- 1 set of 15 reps+ rolling static partials
Do a set of 15 reps in the barbell squat going below parallel. Pause for one second at the bottom and inhale deeply on each rep. After completing 15 reps descend halfway and perform a series of short 6" reps in a pulsing

motion. Pause for several 5- second holds at random points in these short reps. Continue with these reps until your legs are exhausted. Go immediately to the leg extension machine.

Leg extensions- 1 set of 12 reps Superslow+ static holds

Complete a set of 12 reps using the SuperSlow protocol, 10-second positive, or lifting and 4-second lowering phase. After completing these do a series of 10-second static holds with a 10-second rest in-between.

Donkey calf raises- 1 set of 15 reps

Either use a donkey calf machine or have a partner sit on your back while leaning over parallel to the floor, hands and arms resting on a flat bench that is waist high. Place the balls of your feet on a block of wood and lower your heels to the floor. Raise them up as high as you can and flex your calf muscles as hard as you can. Repeat. At the end of the set do a series of short pulsing burn reps until unable to move your muscles at all.

Routine#3

Hack machine squats- 1 set of 12 reps+ negative-accentuated reps+ static holds

Load the machine with a weight that maximizes your efforts at 12 reps. After completing those push yourself to the top of the movement and resist the negative with your left leg only. Press yourself up with both legs and resist with your right leg only. Continue alternating your legs in this fashion until it becomes impossible to control the downward movement. Finally, do a series of 10-second holds with a 5 second rest period in-between. Try and complete a total of 6 of these.

Leg extensions- 1 set of negative-only reps+ static holds

Select a weight that is 40% heavier than you normally use in this exercise. Have your partner lift the machine arms to the fully extended position. After your assistant transfers the resistance to your legs resist the weight as it descends to a count of 8. Continue until you are unable to control the downward movement safely. Increase the weight slightly and extend the machine arms stopping at the ¾ mark. Hold the weight for 10 seconds. As the weight begins to descend have your partner return the weight to the hold start point and hold the weight for as long as you can. Repeat this one more time before reducing the weight and continuing the holds for several more times before ending the set.

Leg curls- 1 set of 15 reps+ partial burn reps

Use a standing, seated or lying leg curl machine with a moderate weight selected. After completing 15 reps do a series of short "burn" reps.

Seated calf machine- 1 set of 15 reps to failure

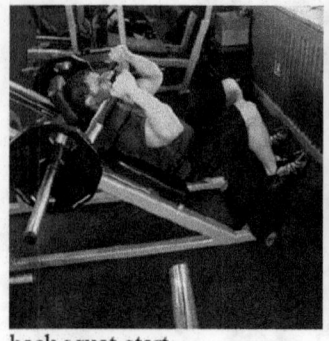 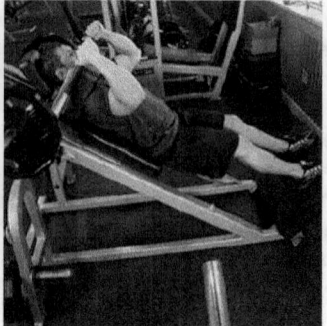

hack squat-start   finish

Back

Routine#1
Machine pullovers- 1 set of 12 reps+ forced reps+ negative reps
Complete a set of 12 reps then have an assistant help you by giving you just
enough help to complete 3 additional reps. The best way to do this is to
place two fingers on the machine arm and as you hit the sticking point apply
pressure to help you complete the rep. After the forced reps have your
assistant lift the arms to the full positive position then transition the weight
to you in a smooth fashion. Resist the weight as it lowers to a count of 8.
Repeat until you can't control the downward movement safely.

Dumbbell Rows- 1 set of 8 negative only reps
Use a pair of dumbbells that are 40% heavier than you typically use for this
exercise. Jerk them up with a cheat motion to use mostly momentum to lift
the weights. Resist them on the way down as you count to 8. Repeat until
unable to control the descent of the weights safely.

Back machine extensions- 1 set of 12 reps + burn reps
Select a moderate weight that allows muscular failure at 12 reps.
After completing 12 reps do a series of burn reps until unable to move the
arms of the machine.

Routine#2
Deadlifts- 1 set of 10 reps
Use a pair of dumbbells or a barbell with a moderate weight. Use a stance
that is slightly wider than shoulder width and hold the barbell or dumbbells
with a cross grip, bend your legs and squat down. Keep your back straight
and pull the bar up as you straighten your legs and bend backward. Repeat
for 10 reps until muscular failure is achieved. Do a series of pulsing "burn"
reps until unable to move the bar.

Straight-arm pulldown- 1 set of 10 reps+ forced reps+ static holds
Attach a double rope handle to the top pulley of a cable machine. If you
don't have a rope handle a medium width straight bar is fine. Select a

moderate weight on the stack. Keeping your arms locked straight in front of you, pull the handle down to your thighs. After completing these have your assistant give you just enough pressure on the bar to allow you to complete 3 additional reps. Increase the weight on the stack and do 4, 10-second holds at the point of full extension. Rest for 5 seconds between holds.

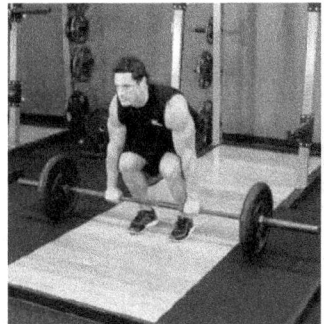 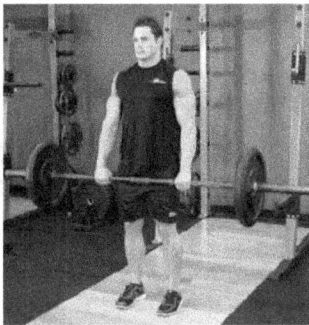

deadlift-start   finish

Routine#3
Machine pullovers- 1 set of 8 reps+ forced reps+ negative reps
Complete a set of 8 reps to failure. Have your partner assist you in performing 4 forced reps. After increasing the weight on the stack have your assistant lift the machine's arms into the bottom position and transfer the weight to you. Resist the motion of the arms to a count of 8 as the weight stack is lowered.
Pulldowns with palms facing each other- 1 set of 10 reps+ forced reps+ static holds
Complete a set of 10 reps to failure. Have a partner help you complete an additional 4 reps. Finally, increase the weight and hold the weight at the point of full contraction for 10 seconds. Rest 5 seconds then do another 10 second hold. Continue until you have completed 6 such holds.
Roman chair hyperextensions- 1 set of 15 reps
Place your feet under the foot anchors on a roman chair bench, lying face down on the bench. Inhale and lower yourself down to as near the bottom. Exhale as you extend yourself up and contract your lower back muscles. Repeat for a total of 15 reps to failure. If you need to add weight, hold a plate behind your head.

It is very important to balance both the strength and muscle tone between your abdominals and your lower back to avoid injuries. If one is dominant over the other injuries could develop due to the superior strength of the other. Hyperextensions and a lower back machine are excellent strengthening tools for the lower back area.

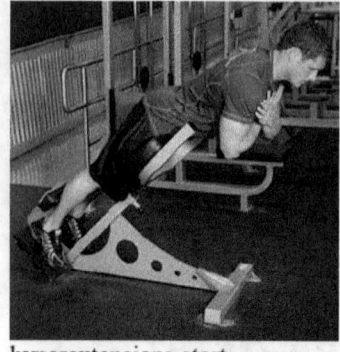 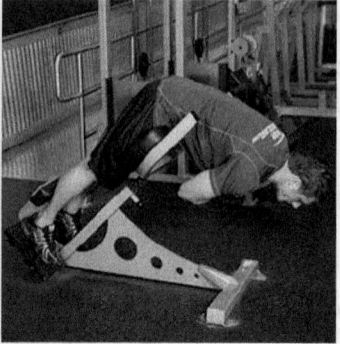

hyperextensions-start   finish

Chest

Routine#1
Incline Dumbbell flyes- 1 set of 10 reps+ forced reps
Lie on an inclined bench while holding two dumbbells off to the side of your chest, arms in a circular arc. Lift the dumbbells in a circular motion as you exhale and stop at the point before they touch. Hold them for 1 second before returning them to the beginning.
Have your partner give you just enough assistance to allow you to complete an additional 4 forced reps. Your partner then assists you in getting the weights up to the top of the movement. Resist the downward movement of the weights to a count of 8. Repeat until you can't control the downward movement safely.
Decline bench presses- 1 set of 8 reps + forced reps+ negative reps
Complete a set of 8 reps. Have your partner assist you in completing an additional 4 forced reps. Your partner then lifts the bar into position and transfers the weight to you. Resist the weight of the bar as it descends to a count of 8. Terminate the set when you are unable to safely control the downward movement of the bar.

Routine#2
Seated dip machine- 1 set of 8 reps+ forced reps+ burn reps
Lean forward in the machine to focus effort on the chest muscles. After completing a set of 8 reps do 4 forced reps with the assistance of a training partner. After finishing the forced reps do a series of 6-inch pulsing reps until unable to move the machine arms.
Cable crossovers- 1 set of 12 reps+ burn reps in each zone
Set the pulleys so they are in the middle position on both sides of the machine and select a moderate weight. Grab the handles and bring them in front of your chest crossing the handles using an arcing motion. At the end

of the set do a series of short-range burn reps in each zone. The best way to do this is to divide the exercise into three zones, upper 3rd, middle 3rd, and last 3rd.

Routine#3
Machine flat bench press- 1 set of pyramid static holds
Set the weight at a moderate weight and press the machine arms to the point near lockout and hold for 10 seconds. Rest for 5 seconds and do another 10 second hold after increasing the weight slightly. Continue until you hit a weight that you can barely hold for 10 seconds. Work your way down the weight stack doing maximum resistance 10 second holds.

Incline machine bench press- 1 set of 12 negatives+ forced reps
Select a weight that is 40% heavier than you typically use in this exercise. Have your assistant lift the handles of the machine to the top and resist the weight on the way down to a count of 8. Repeat for a total of 12 negatives. If you need to reduce the weight after a few reps do so. After completing these do 4 forced reps with a maximum weight that allows you to barely complete the reps with the assistance of your partner.

Shoulders

Routine#1
Seated lateral machine raises- 1 set of 10 reps+ forced reps+ negatives
Complete 10 reps to failure with a moderate weight and after that 4 forced reps with a weight that barely allows you to complete the reps. Do 6 negative-only reps to finish out the set.

Routine#2
Machine presses- 1 set of 12 partial reps in zones+ forced reps+ static holds
Divide the movement into 3 zones. Do 3 reps in each of the zones to failure. With the assistance of a partner complete 4 full forced reps with a maximum weight that barely allows completion of the reps.
Select a maximum weight and hold the handles in the top position for 20 seconds. Repeat by reducing the weight and holding the handles for 20 seconds. Continue in this way until completing a total of 8 static holds.

Routine#3
Standing side/front dumbbell lateral raises- up and down the weight rack
Begin with a moderate weight and complete 10 reps in the side lateral raise, reduce the weight and do a set of 10 front lateral raises. Continue moving up the stack until hitting a maximum weight in each exercise then work your way down the stack until you at near or at the lightest pair of dumbbells.

Arms

Routine#1
Dumbbell curls- 1 set of 10 reps omni-contraction+ forced reps+ static holds

Curl the weights up and lower them 1/3rd of the way and hold for 5 seconds. Lower them to mid-point and hold for 5 seconds. Lower them to the bottom and hold for 5 seconds. Repeat. After completing these, do a series of 4 forced reps with a maximum weight. To complete the set, do 8, 10-second static holds with maximum weight.

Seated tricep machine extensions- 1 set of 10 reps SuperSlow+ forced reps+ negatives

Use a weight that is 30% lighter than you normally use in this exercise. Press the arms of the machine to full extension using a rep cadence of 10 seconds positive and 4 seconds negative. After completing 10 reps do 4 forced reps in the same SuperSlow cadence with the assistance of a partner. To finish the set, have a partner press the arms to the end position and resist the weight to a count of 8. Repeat for a total of 6 negatives.

Routine#2
Rope curls- 1 set of 10 reps+ forced reps+ negatives

Attach a double rope handle to the middle pulley of a cable machine and select a moderate weight. Curl the rope handle into your chin. Pause for one second then return. Complete 10 reps followed by 4 forced reps and 5 negative reps.

Dumbbell overhead press- 1 set of 8 reps+ negatives

Complete 8 reps followed by 8 negative reps with the help of a partner.

Routine#3
Machine curls- 1 set of 12 negatives+ burn reps

Complete 12 negative reps either one arm at a time or both arms with the help of an assistant. After completing these finish the set by doing a series of short-range burn reps until unable to move the curling handle at all.

Close-grip bench press- 1 set of 12 negatives+ 6 rest-pause reps

Use an 18" wide grip. Using a maximum weight do 12 negative reps. After completing those press the bar up for one maximum rep, rest 10 seconds then repeat. Continue until you have completed a total of 8 rest-pause reps. Reduce the weight as necessary to allow you to use good form.

Abdominals

Since we aren't looking to build too much muscle in the abdominal region, we will use a standard routine. Use a high-moderate rep count with added weight as necessary. Train all parts of the region including the upper and lower abs and side Serratus areas.

Routine#1

Ab crunches- 1 set of 15 reps
Use a machine if one is available. If not add weight via a weight plate held at your chest.

Leg raises on bench- 1 set of 15 or more reps
Lie flat on a weight bench with your legs together. You may bend your legs if you are unable to do leg raises with your legs straight. Using all muscle power and no momentum, lift your legs up until they are straight overhead. Repeat for as many reps as you can.

Side bends with dumbbells- 1 set of 15 reps each side
Standing straight, hold a dumbbell in each hand at your side. Bend to the left as far down as is comfortable. Reverse direction and bend to the right as far as you can. Continue until you have completed 15 reps per side.

Routine#2

Ab wheel contractions- 1 set of as many reps as you can
Kneel on the floor and hold an ab wheel in front of you on the floor. Keep your arms slightly bent and extend yourself out in front as far as you can. Using your stomach muscles, and not your legs, pull yourself back in. Repeat for as many reps as you can.

Hanging leg raises- 1 set of as many reps as you can
Hang from a chinning bar with your legs hanging down. Bring your knees up as high as you can. Repeat for as many reps as you can.

This concludes our training routines using the ultra- high intensity protocol. This is a very advanced training strategy and should not be used until you have been training with standard HIT, high intensity routines for at least six months. It is very important to train with maximum intensity when using this protocol because you have a very limited amount of sets to use to stimulate muscle growth. The idea with this system is to maximize the effort put forth into a very small (1-2 total sets per body part) set count and provide the most muscle growth stimulus with the minimal amount of training. This prevents overtraining and is ideal for instigating muscle growth.

Mike Mentzer, one of the pioneers of high intensity training, used this system to train seven-time Mr. Olympia, Dorian Yates after Mr. Yates had become stale in his training. He contacted Mike and hired him to coach him to his next Mr. Olympia win, which he did. Mike expressed to Dorian that he needed to reduce the volume of his training and increase the intensity dramatically. The training routines outlined in this section are indicative of the type of routines Mike used successfully.

Band training

There are many different types of rubber tubes and bands available to train with exclusively or in conjunction with other training apparatus such as machines, free weights and bodyweight exercises. They are rated in pounds of resistance, often using a range from say, 15-30 lbs. of resistance as well as many other combinations. The bands necessarily increase in thickness as they go up in resistance. The resistance tubes are made from surgical tubing while the extra duty bands, commonly used in powerlifting training, are made from thick, flat rubber and resemble a large, heavy-duty rubber band.

I have found bands to be very useful and complementary to my training with both weight machines and free weights. Many of the exercises with bands are very close to dumbbell and cable machine exercises but lend a different feel to the exercises as opposed to the machines. This is great for variation in training because the bands change the action of each exercise. This changes the way the exercises interact with the muscles and helps to stimulate new growth.

There are many ways to use bands in your training. I will outline the ways I have found to be most effective. It is a good idea to obtain a door attachment device so you can use a strong door as an anchor for your bands. If you choose, you may attach the heavy-duty bands to a post or other strong fixture by looping it through itself and holding on to the free end for your exercises.

Action of the bands and tubes

The main reason for the different feel of bands and tubes should be obvious. As you stretch the band during an exercise and it gets longer, the resistance increases at a rapid pace. This is different from all free weight exercises because in free weights the weight resistance remains the same throughout although the angle of movement changes altering the force placed on the muscle.

A weight machine that has a proper cam on it is closer to the feel of a band because the range of motion and variable resistance is more similar to the action of a band although they both arrive at their resistance curves differently. The machine's cam is engineered and built with a variable thickness to it, which changes the amount of force placed on the muscle being trained whereas the band resistance isn't nearly as sophisticated. It merely increases the more you pull, push or twist it because the rubber is being stretched further.

Since there is no weight to the bands and their resistance comes in the form of rubber resistance, gravity and its complications aren't a factor. That is a distinct advantage compared to free weight exercises, such as the barbell curl, where angles and gravity become a real drawback. Using the curl as an example, the lift begins at the bottom where there is little resistance. The bar travels to the midpoint where resistance is highest and ends at the top where virtually all of the resistance has faded. Unfortunately, when the resistance is removed from the exercise so is the benefit. Once you incorporate band training into your routine you will agree that these are really effective tools. Now let's try some routines.

Legs

Band squats- 1 set of 15 reps
Use a heavy resistance band for this exercise. Step on the band with both legs and pull the other end onto your shoulders. Keep your back straight and squat down until your legs are below parallel, breathe deep and press yourself up. Repeat.
Band lunges- 1 set of 12 reps per leg
Use a small band designed to hold both legs together. Begin with both legs side by side. Step forward with your left leg as far as is comfortable and step back. Step forward with your right leg and bring it back. Repeat. This exercise is drastically different than a typical dumbbell or barbell lunge where you take a deep step forward while holding a dumbbell or barbell for resistance. With the band lunge, you are stepping forward against a strong resistance, which focuses a lot of the effort on your hips, which allows you to strengthen the hip area.
One-legged band squats- 1 set of 15 reps
Step into a heavy band with one foot and place the other end over the shoulder on the same side as the leg you are training. Squat down while stabilizing yourself with your other hand as far as you can and return. Repeat for 15 reps on your left leg before changing to your right leg.

Bands in conjunction with traditional equipment

Leg extensions- 1 set of 15 reps
These are performed in the normal way. Make sure to get a really good contraction at the top of the exercise. Do this set to failure.
Band squats- 1 set of 12 reps
Complete this exercise as described in the two-legged squat above. Go as near to failure as you can.
Machine leg presses- 1 set of 8 reps+ one-legged negative reps
Get a full range of motion on these to get the full effect of this exercise.

After finishing the 8 reps, press the footplate up with both legs and resist the plate back down with your left leg only. Repeat this and resist the footplate with your right leg only. Continue alternating like this until you are unable to safely control the downward movement.

Seated calf raises- 1 set of 15 reps to failure
Use a moderate weight on the machine. Place your feet on the block and let your heels get a good stretch as they almost touch the floor. Lift the machine arm up as high as you can and flex your calves hard. Repeat.

Chest

Band crossovers- 1 set of 12 reps
Use one or two bands for this exercise. Attach each band to a strong support, either a doorway via a connector or tie it to a post by looping one end through the other. Stand next to the band and keep your arms slightly bent. Bring the band across your chest until it is past the center and tense your chest muscles hard. Repeat.

Band chest presses- 1 set of 8 reps
Attach a strong band to a support and brace your back against it. Grab the band with both hands and press it out in front of you. Make sure that your elbows are pointing out to your side parallel to the floor. You should get a really great contraction at the end position. Repeat. This exercise can be done with one or two arms at a time.

Band upward crossovers- 1 set of 8 reps
Attach a band low on a support. Grab the end while keeping your arms bent, and bring it up diagonally across your chest. If the resistance is heavy and you push yourself you will get a very strong contraction. Repeat. Once you complete 8 reps with that side change arms and train the other side.

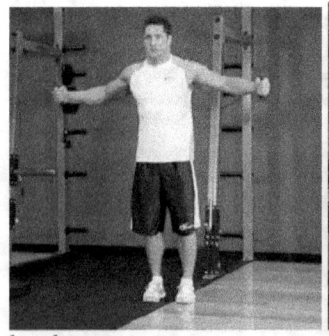 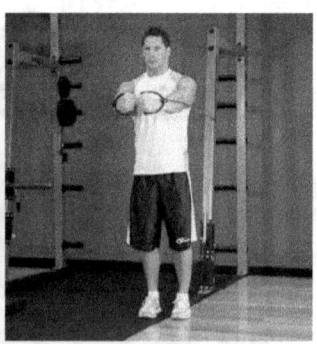

band crossovers-start   finish

Bands in conjunction with traditional equipment

Band crossovers- 1 set of 12 reps
Inclined bench press with barbell – 1 set of 6 reps+ 3 forced reps at the end of the set
Seated dip machine- 1 set of 8 reps+ 3 forced reps at the end of the set

Back

Band rows 1-arm- 1 set of 6 reps
Step on the end of a heavy resistance band. Grab the other end and row it to you abdomen while bending your upper body parallel to the floor. Repeat. After finishing 6 reps change arms and do 6 reps with that side.
Band straight-arm pulldowns- 1 set of 10 reps
Attach a band overhead, and using a straight-arm grip, pull the band down with both arms. Contract your lats hard at the bottom before returning. Repeat.
Machine pullovers- 1 set of 10 reps+ 4 forced reps
Using a pullover machine do a set of 10 reps followed by 4 forced reps

Bands in conjunction with traditional equipment

Reverse flyes- 1 set of 12 reps
Sit facing in on a pek dek machine or a reverse flye machine. Grab the handles, keeping your arms slightly bent, and bring the handles back using an arcing motion. The movement resembles a pek flye movement just in reverse. Use good form with no jerking motion.
Band straight-arm pulldowns- 1 set of 10 reps
Attach a medium band overhead. Grab the end with both hands and pull it straight down keeping your arms locked out in front of you. Complete 10 reps.
Incline dumbbell rows- 1 set of 6 reps
Use an inclined bench for this exercise. Using a shoulder-width grip, pull the bar up to the bench and return.

Shoulders

Band shoulder front lateral raises- 1 set of 12 reps
Use a light resistance band for this exercise in the beginning.
Step on one end and grab the other end with an overhand grip. With a slight bend in your arm, raise the band straight up to a point slightly higher than your shoulders and return. Complete a total of 12 reps then switch arms and repeat.
Band bent-over lateral raises- 1 set of 12 reps
Use the same band for this exercise as the one you used in the previous exercise. Bend over until you are parallel to the floor. Step on one end of the

band and grip the other with an overhand grip. Bend your arms slightly and raise the band until your arm is parallel to the floor. Repeat. Complete a total of 12 reps then switch arms and repeat.

Band presses- 1 set of 8 reps
Use a heavy resistance band. Step on the band with both feet and grab the other end with both hands. Press the band up to the pre-lockout position. Repeat.

Bands in conjunction with traditional equipment

Dumbbell side lateral raises- 1 set of 10 reps
Use a pair of dumbbells for this exercise. Stand straight while holding a dumbbell at each side. Keeping your arms slightly bent, raise the weights out to the side until they are slightly higher than shoulder height. Lower the weights then repeat.

Machine press behind neck- 1 set of 6 rest-pause reps+ negative reps
Select a heavy weight that is near your 1RM in this lift. Lift the machine handle up to the pre-lockout position and return. Rest for 10 seconds then repeat. After a couple of reps you will need to reduce the weight. With the assistance of a partner, do a series of negative reps until you are unable to control the descent of the weight.

Band upright rows- 1 set of 12 reps
Select a medium resistance band. Step on the one end with both feet and grip the other end with both hands. Bend your arms and lift the band straight up until it is at shoulder height. Return. Repeat for a total of 12 reps.

Arms

Band two-handed curls- 1 set of 6 reps
Use a medium resistance band for this exercise. Step on one end of the band with both feet and grab the other with both hands. Keeping your elbows locked at your sides, curl the band up to shoulder height and return. Repeat for a total of 6 reps.

Band overhead curls one-handed- 1 set of 10 reps
Attach a band overhead. Grab the band with one hand after lying on a flat bench. Curl the band down to your forehead and flex your biceps muscle hard before return to the top. Repeat for a total of 10 reps before switching hands and training that arm.

Band concentration curls- 1 set of 10 reps
Attach a band to the floor. Bend over and place the arm being trained on the same side knee. Grab the band and curl it up to your chin and return. Complete a total of 10 reps before switching to train the other arm.

Bands in conjunction with traditional equipment

Incline dumbbell curls- 1 set of 12 reps
Sit on an incline bench and curl a dumbbell up to chin level and return. Do a total of 12 reps before switching hands and training the other arm.

One-handed band high curl- 1 set of 8 reps
Attach a band at shoulder height to a firm door attachment or some other firm surface. Stand sideways to the band and grab the end with one hand. Lift your arm straight out from your shoulder. Curl the band into your body and flex your biceps muscle hard before returning. Complete a total of 8 reps before training the other arm.

Barbell preacher curl- 1 set of 12 reps rolling static partials+ negatives
Place your upper arms on a preacher bench. Get a good stretch at the beginning of the rep and curl the weight all the way up to your chin. Let the weight down part of the way and do a static hold for 5 reps. Do a few burn reps at this point then move the bar up slightly to a random position and do some more burn reps and then a 5 second static hold.

Continue doing full and partial reps and static holds. This is my rolling static partial technique, which is very effective due to the fact that you are doing partials, static holds and burn reps, all in the same set. Once you are experienced with this technique you will be able to maximize its effectiveness. Complete the set by doing 4 negative reps with the assistance of a training partner.

Band tricep pushdowns- 1 set of 8 reps+ static holds
Attach a band overhead. Grab the bottom end with both hands and push it straight down. Complete 8 reps with each rep containing a 10 second static hold within it.

Seated band tricep extensions- 1 set of 10 reps+ burn reps
Attach a band to the floor while sitting on a flat bench. Using both hands grab the band behind you and extend it overhead. Make sure to keep both elbows firmly against the sides of your head during the exercise.

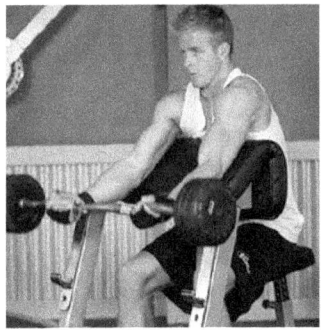 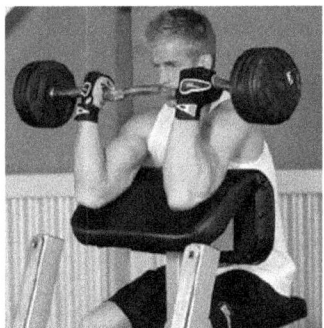

preacher curl-start   finish

Bands in conjunction with traditional equipment

Band angled extensions- 1 set of 10 reps+ static holds
Attach a band at a level just below shoulder height. Brace yourself against
the band, grab the other end of the band with both hands and press it
outward at a downward angle. Do a total of 10 reps with each rep having a
10 second static hold in it.
Machine triceps extensions- 1 set of 12 reps rest-pause
Select a weight that is just less than your 1RM. Press the handles to full
extension and return. Rest 10 seconds then press for an additional rep.
Reduce the weight slightly then repeat. Reduce the weight as necessary to
complete 12 max reps.

Now that I've outlined some band-only and band/traditional equipment
training routines, I'll list exercises that can be done with bands:

- Running in place – Attach a band around your waist after anchoring it
  to a wall behind you. Run in place while pulling forward against the
  resistance of the band. Use a strong band that is capable of holding
  you back while stretching a normal amount to avoid stressing it.
- Band squats- Do these one-legged or with both legs. To do the one-
  legged variety, Step on one end of a heavy-duty band and place the
  other end over your shoulder of the same side a s the leg to be trained.
  Stabilize yourself by holding on to a chair or pole and squat down as
  far as you can. Inhale deeply and press yourself up with your leg.
  For the two-legged squat, step on one end of a band with both feet and
  place the other end on both shoulders in front of you. Execute the
  exercise in the same way as one-legged squats.
- Leg lunges- Attach a small band around the outside of both legs at calf
  level. Step forward with your left leg as far as you can. You will be
  very limited in the distance you can step due to the size of the band in
  comparison to the dumbbell variety. Bring your leg back and repeat the
  movement with your right leg.
- Leg extensions- Attach a band to a wall. Place your foot through
  the other end while bracing your back against the wall. Extend your leg
  forward in a motion similar to machine leg extensions and return to the
  floor.
- Ab crunches- Attach a band near the floor. Hold the band behind your
  head with both hands and perform a crunch. In most cases it will be
  necessary to use a low-tension band.
- Side bends- Step on the end of a band with your left foot and hold the
  other end with your left hand. Keep your arm straight and bend to your

right as far as you can. Do a series of reps before switching to your other side.

- Stiff-legged deadlifts- Stand on a heavy tension band with both feet, with a shoulder-width stance. Hold the band with both hands in an overhand grip. Keeping your legs locked, stand up and back slightly.
- Deadlifts- Position yourself like you did in the stiff-legged deadlift. Bend your legs as you squat down to grab the band with both hands. Bring yourself up like a standard deadlift.
- Band crossovers- Attach a band low, medium or high height on a pole or other fixture. Hold the band with one hand, and using an arcing motion, bring it across your chest in front of you. Alternately you can use two bands and train both sides of your chest at the same time.
- Chest press- This is a bench press with bands. Because of the versatility of the bands you can train one side of your chest by doing one-arm presses or both sides by using either two bands with one arm on each side or one band for a two-handed press.
- Angled-up pec lift- Grab a band with one hand. Keeping your arm slightly bent lift the band across your chest at an upward angle.
- Stiff-arm pulldown- Attach a band overhead. Hold the band with both hands while keeping your arms locked straight and pull the band down to your lower thighs.
- One-arm or two-arm low row- Attach a band to the floor, grab the band and row it to your lower abs.
- Middle level row- Attach a band to the wall or other fixture at mid-level. Using one or two arms, pull the band to your chest.
- Pulldown- Attach a band overhead. Pull the band down to your chest.
- Deadlifts- This was explained above.
- Stiff-legged deadlifts- Explained above
- Curls- Explained above
- Concentration curls- Attach a band on the floor. Bend over and place your elbow on your knee on the same side as the arm you're training. Curl the band to your chin.

There are many additional exercises available to get yourself fit, strong and muscular if desired but these are most of the standard exercises.

One of the things I really like about training with bands in conjunction with free weights and weight machines is the ability to train hard with the weight machine and follow that with a set of a band exercise and work the exercise through standard reps, partial reps or rolling static partial reps.

As you pull or push further on a band the resistance level increases, which is ideal because the point of maximum contraction is almost always at the endpoint of an exercise. This is demonstrated by leg extensions, where the leg muscles are maxed out at the fully extended position. So get a good set of training bands and some resistance tubes and add them to your training equipment inventory.

Types of Bands
- Power Bands
- Resistance Tubes
- Flat Bands

Kettlebells

Kettlebells have been around for well over 150 years and were the staple of training for many strongmen of yesteryear. Even though they are somewhat similar to dumbbells, they have some unique properties to them giving trainees a tool that is very capable of training the entire body with not only standard exercises but also many exercises that are unique to kettlebells.

A kettlebell looks like a hunk of rounded steel with a handle on top, which is basically what it is. Standard kettlebells have a rounded handle on top, which gives one the ability to use it with one or both hands. A newer style of kettlebell, called a competition kettlebell has a square handle with rounded edges at the top. They have the same dimensions regardless of the weight of the kettlebell. This is to balance them during competitive kettlebell lifting competitions.

Some benefits of kettlebell training include:

- Full-body conditioning-The body works as one synergistic unit linked together

- Big results by spending less time in the gym- kettlebell training involves multiple muscle groups at once

- Increased resistance to injury

- The ability to work aerobically and anaerobically at the same time.

- Improved mobility and range of motion

- Increased strength

- Enhanced performance in athletics and everyday functioning

- Weight loss-One university study found that kettlebell training burned an average of 20 calories per minute

Now lets outline some kettlebell training programs and exercises for you to train with. As a beginner do a total of one round of each exercise with a one-minute rest between exercises. As you advance, shorten the rest periods to 30 seconds and add an additional round of the exercises. Finally, complete three rounds of each exercise with minimal or no rest between exercises.

The advantage of kettlebell training is that it is very functional-in other words- it uses your entire body's muscle groups for the majority of the exercises. This builds co-ordination and a high amount of conditioning and strength. This helps get you ready for both everyday life and any sports you may engage in.

Beginner

Two-handed kettlebell swing- Grab a kettlebell with both hands while standing in a wide squat position. Using muscle power only, swing the weight up until it is overhead and return. Your arms should be locked straight throughout. The picture demonstrates a one-handed swing, which is a good alternative to the two-handed version.

Two-handed kettlebell reverse lunge- Hold a kettlebell of the same weight in each hand at arms length by your side. Step back as far as you can with your left leg and squat down on it. Return and step back with your right leg and squat down on it.

Kettlebell squat- Hold a kettlebell against your chest with both hands. With a stance that is slightly wider than shoulder width, squat all of the way down until you are about 10 inches off the floor. Push yourself up to the standing position and repeat.

Kettlebell clean and press- Clean a pair of kettlebells from the floor to your shoulders and press them overhead while squatting down part way.

One- hand kettlebell 'round the worlds- Stand erect while holding a kettlebell in your right hand. Circle the kettlebell, using a left circular motion around the front of your body, while handing the weight off to your left hand. Bring the kettlebell around the back of your body with your left hand and hand it to your right hand. Continue moving the kettlebell around your body in this way.

Ab crunches- Assume a crunch position on the floor with your knees up while holding a kettlebell behind your head. Crunch your abs until you have a strong contraction. Repeat

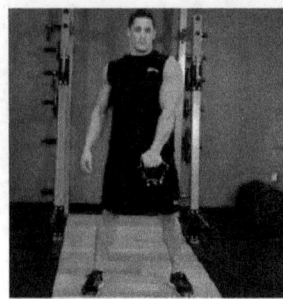
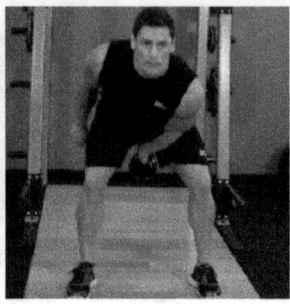

kettlebell swing one-handed-start   bottom

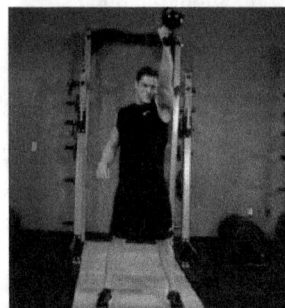

end

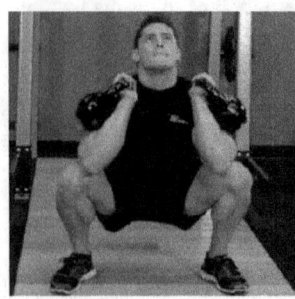
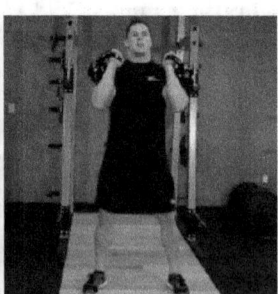

kettlebell squat-start   finish

Advanced routine#1

One- hand kettlebell swing with left rotation- Hold a kettlebell in your left hand while crouched down in a squat position. Keeping your arm straight bring the weight up in front of you and arc it to the left bringing it down to the left of your left leg. Bring the kettlebell up overhead and let it come down to the beginning position. Repeat.

One- hand kettlebell swing with right rotation- Same as above except reverse directions and use your right hand and do a right rotation.

Two-hand kettlebell swing- Same as the kettlebell swing in the beginner's workout.

Two-hand kettlebell squat- Same as in the beginner's workout.

Two- hand kettlebell reverse lunge- Same as the beginner's workout.

Two hand kettlebell clean and press- Clean two kettlebells to your shoulders with one kettlebell in each hand. Press the kettlebells overhead.

Two-hand kettlebell high pulls- Bend over at your waist and grab a kettlebell. Straighten up at the same time you pull the kettlebell up to chin level. This movement resembles a "good morning" exercise and upright row exercise combined.

One –hand kettlebell cross-chest angles- Hold a kettlebell in your left hand by your side. Lift the kettlebell up and across your chest, ending in front of your right pectoral muscle. After a series of reps, switch hands and train your right side.

Kettlebell ab crunches- Same as the beginner's workout.

Advanced routine#2

Two-hand kettlebell swing- Same as the beginner's workout.

Two-hand kettlebell squat/press- Clean a kettlebell to your shoulders with both hands. Squat down as far as you can using a stance slightly wider than shoulder width and press the kettlebell overhead. As you come up from the squat lower the weight back to your shoulders. Set the kettlebell back on the floor. Repeat for the desired amount of reps.

Two-hand kettlebell clean and press- Same as the beginner's workout.

Two-hand kettlebell snatch-Clean the kettlebell in one motion all the way overhead. Squat down "under" the kettlebell as necessary to allow you to clean it and stand up once the kettlebell is overhead.

Two-hand kettlebell deadlift- Use one kettlebell in each hand and do a standard deadlift. Use a stance that is slightly wider than shoulder width.

One-hand kettlebell get-up- Lay on the floor while holding a kettlebell on your chest. Sit up and position your left leg to begin lifting yourself up. At the same time begin lifting yourself up with your free arm. Continue to lift yourself up with your legs and free arm being careful to avoid dropping the kettlebell on yourself.

One-arm kettlebell row- Brace your free arm on a dumbbell rack or bench. Row the kettlebell up to your lower abdomen with one arm. Switch arms and train the other side.

One-hand tricep kickback- Hold a kettlebell in your left hand while leaning forward. Brace yourself by holding onto a bench or rack with your right hand. Press the kettlebell back as far as you can while keeping your upper arm stationary against your body. Flex your tricep muscle hard at the point of full contraction to activate the maximum amount of fibers.

Two-hand kettlebell ab crunches- As explained previously.

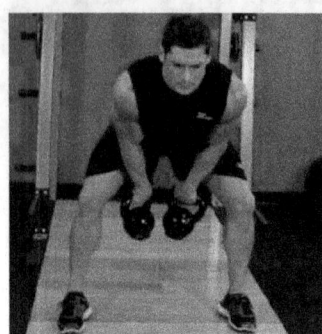 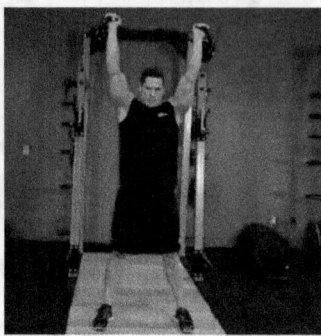

kettlebell snatch-start   finish

Advanced routine#3

Two-hand kettlebell squat and press- Explained previously.
Two-hand kettlebell clean and press- Explained previously.
Two-hand kettlebell deadlift- Explained previously.
Two-hand kettlebell reverse lunge- Explained previously.
One-hand kettlebell figure 8's- Stand erect and hold a kettlebell in your right hand. Move the kettlebell around your body in a figure 8 outline by putting the kettlebell through your legs and moving it in a circular motion around your hips.
One-hand kettlebell concentration curl- Perform this in the same way that you do a dumbbell concentration curl.
One-hand tricep kickback- Explained previously.
Two-hand incline bench ab sit-ups- Use a kettlebell to add weight to standard incline sit-ups.

Advanced routine#4

Two-hand kettlebell deadlift- Explained previously.
Two-hand kettlebell row- This is the same as the one hand kettlebell row except it is performed either with two hands on one kettlebell or with a kettlebell in each hand.

Two-hand chest press- This is the same as a two-hand dumbbell bench press except using two kettlebells.
Two-hand kettlebell clean and press- Explained previously.
Two-hand kettlebell front lateral raises- This is the same as dumbbell lateral raises except with kettlebells.
Two-hand kettlebell upright rows- Same as dumbbell upright rows except with kettlebells.
One-hand kettlebell curls- This is the same as dumbbell curls except with kettlebells.
Two-hand kettlebell tricep overhead extensions- This is the same as dumbbell overhead tricep extensions except with kettlebells.
Leg raises- Lie on the floor with your legs together. Raise your legs until they are overhead. Lower them and repeat.

Medicine Ball Exercise

Medicine balls have been used in boxers' training throughout boxing history. They were dropped on a boxer's stomach to toughen up his ab muscles against punching attacks during a match but today they have become popular and many people train with them, especially crossfitters. The reason is they are very effective and easy to use.

There are many different types such as leather, rubber, special coated grip and slam balls. The latter is so named because the ball is repeatably thrown, or slammed against the wall or floor. This is done to give the user powerful explosive strength, which helps certain athletes train for their sports. For exercisers that are not athletes routines will include side bends, squats, presses, slams and other exercises.

Medicine balls are available in different weights ranging from 3-150 pounds. The important thing is to use a weight that taxes you but isn't a severe strain to use. If you are able to use good form in your exercises, you are probably using the correct weighted ball.

Power is the result of the combination of speed and strength. The ability to generate maximum power, developed through functional training, is a key to being a successful athlete. It also helps an individual with everyday activities and is important if you become involved in a severe stressful situation.

The muscle fibers responsible for fast, explosive movements are the high threshold motor units, which are muscle fibers that have the ability to contract very fast and explosively. This ability is also known as neuromuscular efficiency and is enhanced with explosive medicine ball training.

Now, lets take a look at some great training routines for you to use. We'll begin with a good basic routine then progress to an intermediate and finally an advanced one.

Basic medicine ball workout
- Medicine ball squats- Hold the ball overhead and stand shoulder width apart. Squat down as far as you can and return to upright position. Keep your back straight throughout.
- Medicine ball overhead throws- Squat down into a low crouch while holding the ball with both hands. Stand up straight and throw the ball overhead as high as you can in a rapid motion.
- Medicine ball chest throws- Stand upright while holding a medicine ball with both hands. Throw the ball as hard as you can against a wall or to a partner in front of you. Catch the ball when it returns to you.
- Medicine ball lateral throws- Stand next to a wall, facing it sideways about 10' away. Throw the ball sideways at the wall and catch it when it comes back. After doing a series of reps change sides
- Medicine ball swings- Stand with a stance that is shoulder-width apart. Hold a medicine ball with both hands and swing it down between your legs as you crouch down slightly. Swing the ball up overhead using no momentum.

Do one series of all of the exercises using a rep count of 10 for each. Rest one minute between exercises. This workout trains your entire body and builds co-ordination and functional strength.

Intermediate medicine ball workout
- Medicine ball leg lunges- Hold the medicine ball with both hands. Take a deep step forward with your left leg while descending into a low stance over your outstretched leg. Push yourself back up with your outstretched leg and repeat the movement with your right leg. Continue alternating legs until the desired rep count is achieved.
- Medicine ball shoulder press- Stand upright while holding the ball at chest level with both hands. Press the ball overhead and return. You can use a heavy ball to make this harder or do this one arm at a time.
- Medicine ball chest throws- Stand upright while holding a medicine ball with both hands. Throw the ball as hard as you can against a wall or to a partner in front of you. Catch the ball when it returns to you.
- Figure 8- Stand with feet about shoulder-width apart. Hold onto a medicine ball with both hands to one side of the head, with arms fully extended. Slowly move the medicine ball in a fluid, controlled motion, forming the figure 8. Repeat 8-10 reps through clockwise,

then switch directions. This one can be deceivingly tiring, so try it with a lighter ball first.

- Medicine ball rows- Lean over until your upper body is perpendicular to the ground while holding the ball at arms length. Pull the ball up to your chest and return.
- Medicine ball overhead throws- Squat down into a low crouch while holding the ball with both hands. Stand up straight and throw the ball overhead as high as you can in a rapid motion.
- Medicine ball lateral throws- Stand next to a wall, facing it sideways about 10' away. Throw the ball sideways at the wall and catch it when it comes back. After doing a series of reps, change sides.
- Medicine ball swings- Stand with a stance that is shoulder-width apart. Hold a medicine ball with both hands and swing it down between your legs as you crouch down slightly. Swing the ball up overhead using no momentum.

Do a total of 2 circuits of all exercises in the same order. Complete 10 reps per exercise. To progress to an advanced workout, do 3-4 circuits of the intermediate routine in the same order, completing 10 reps per exercise. Rest one minute between circuits.

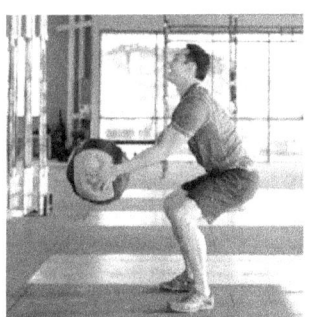 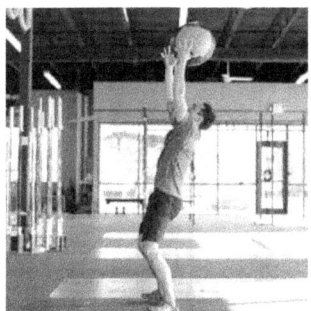

medicine ball overhead throw-start   finish

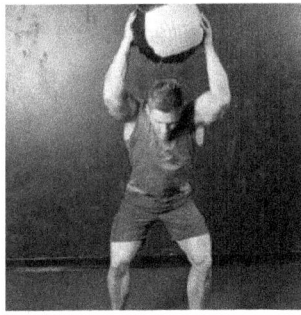 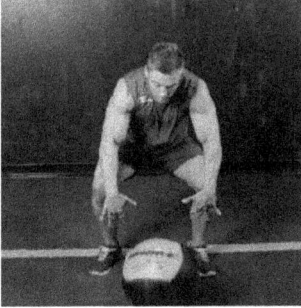

medicine ball slam-start   finish

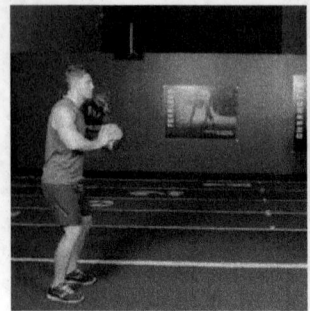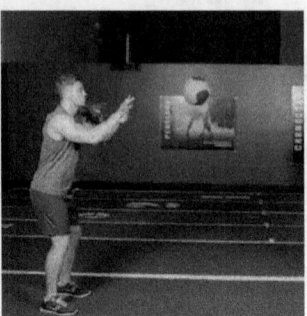

medicine ball chest throw-start   finish

Bodyweight Training

The great thing about bodyweight training is the cost of the equipment needed is extremely low-in most cases it's free! In school we knew these exercises as calisthenics and did them over and over again in gym class.

As soon as we graduated from school we forgot about them and years later many of us began training with weights-both free weights and machines- at a local gym. In most cases trainers focus on machines and free weights and have forgotten how useful and complementary bodyweight exercises are in a training program when used in conjunction with other tools.

Many of these bodyweight exercises are similar to free weight and weight machine exercises in motion but offer the advantage of ability to train away from the gym in the outdoors with no one else around or in a group setting in or outdoors. If you travel often and are unable to get to the gym, this type of training is great because it can be done in the comfort of your hotel room.

Some of the exercises we will be using in this program are various types of pushups, sit-ups, ab crunches, pull-ups, reverse lunges, lunge, deep knee bends, bar dips, burpees, calf raises and hyperextensions. Some of the exercises can be used in conjunction with weights to add resistance to the movements.

This training is very effective for losing fat and gaining muscle and some form of training can be used by almost everybody of any age and health level. These are also great for the training of athletes of all sports including bodybuilders in or out of competition.

In the beginning we will begin with one circuit or giant set of all of the exercises with a rest period between them and work up to a circuit with zero rest between exercises.

The following is a list of the exercises we will be using. After you become familiar with this list I will outline several training routines using them.

Inchworm: Stand up tall with your legs straight and let your fingertips touch the floor. Keeping your legs straight (but not locked), slowly lower your torso toward the floor and walk your hands forward. Once in a push-up position, start taking tiny steps so your feet meet your hands. Continue for 4-6 reps.

Mountain Climber: Starting on your hands and knees, bring your left foot forward directly under your chest while straightening your right leg. Keep your hands on the ground and abs tight, and jump while switching legs. Your left leg should now be extended behind your body with your right knee forward.

Burpees: One of the more effective bodyweight exercises, start out in a low squat position with your hands on the floor. Next, kick your feet back to a push-up position, complete one push-up, then immediately return your feet to the squat position. Leap up as high as possible before squatting and moving back into the push-up portion of the show.

Plank: Lie face down with your forearms and hands clasped. Extend your legs behind your body and rise up on your toes. Keeping your back straight, tighten your core and hold the position for 30-60 seconds or as long as you can.

Lunge: Stand with your hands on your hips and feet hip-width apart. Step forward with your right leg and slowly lower your body until your right knee is close to touching the floor and bent at least 90 degrees. Return to the starting position and repeat with your left leg.

Reverse lunge- This is the same as the lunge except you step backward with your leg instead of forward.

Deep knee bend- Stand with your feet parallel. Slowly start to descend by bending your hips and knees until your thighs are parallel to the floor. If you can go lower safely, do so. Make sure your heels do not rise off the floor. Return to a standing position.

Push-Up: With hands shoulder-width apart, keep your feet together and tighten your mid-section. Bend your elbows until your chest reaches the ground and push back up. Keep your elbows tucked close to your body.

Bar dips- Grab the handles of a set of dip bars and push yourself up to full extension while leaning forward. Lower yourself back down and repeat.

Ab crunches- Lie on the floor facing up. Clench your hands behind your head and keep your knees bent and your feet together. Simultaneously lift your upper body and legs toward each other and flex your ab muscles hard before returning to the start position.

Calf raises- Stand erect on the balls of your feet and lift yourself up as far as you can before returning to the beginning position, lowering yourself as far as you can for a full stretch.

Sit-ups- Lie flat on the floor with your hands clenched together behind your head. Sit up and bring your upper body as far toward your legs as possible. Return to the beginning position. An alternative way to do this exercise is to raise your knees up in a position similar to the ab crunch.

Triceps Dip: Sit near a bench on the floor with knees slightly bent and grab the edge of the bench and straighten your arms. Bend them to a 90-degree angle and straighten again while the heels push towards the floor.

L Seat: Sit with legs extended and feet flexed and place your hands on the floor and slightly round the torso. Lift your hips off the ground and hold for five seconds and release. Repeat!

Hyperextensions- Lie face down on the floor with your hands clasped behind your head. Raise your upper body and legs off the ground at the same time and hold for 10 seconds. Lower them back to the floor and repeat.

Pull-up- Using either a palms facing, pull-up grip, a traditional chin-up or palms facing away grip, pull yourself up to an overhead bar and lower yourself back down. Repeat for as many reps as you can.

Rotational circles- Stand straight with your arms out to your sides parallel with the floor at shoulder height. Begin by rotating your arms in forward circles. After a series of reps, reverse the direction and do a series of reps in that direction.

Workout#1

Deep knee bend
Pull-up
Push-up
Burpee
Plank
Hyperextension

As a beginner, do one cycle of as many reps as you can in each exercise.
As you become more advanced increase the workload to two cycles. Under no circumstances should you ever exceed four cycles.

Workout#2

Leg lunges
Chin-up
Bar dips
Inchworm
Rotational circles
Ab crunches

Same advice as above.

Workout#3

Reverse leg lunges
Push-up
Pull-up
Mountain climber
Plank
Leg raises

Same advice as above.

Workout#4

Deep knee bend
L-seat
Burpee
Hyperextensions
Tricep dip
Ab crunches

Leg raises

Same advice as above.

Some of the exercises such as push-ups, knee bends, tricep dips, pull-ups and bar dips lend themselves well to adding weight via a weight plate or dip belt, if desired, to make the exercises more difficult.

Feel free to come up with new combinations of these exercises but remember these workouts were formulated to train the entire body in the proper order so substitute a leg exercise for another on, etc.

Power Rack Training

While there are many useful tools to train with such as barbells, dumbbells, machines, various bars and attachments, one of the most useful tools for building muscle size and power is the power rack.

Consisting of four upright posts drilled with holes attached to a base on the floor and the ceiling, a power rack is used with a standard or Olympic barbell to safely train in power lifts and other barbell exercises.

Four pins are used to place in the holes to support, or spot the bar if the lifter needs or desires to set the bar down and prevent the bar from traveling above a certain height in the rack.

This can be used to advantage in overcoming so-called "sticking points"- points in barbell lifts where the bar comes to a screeching halt- preventing you from increasing the weight that you are able to lift in a certain exercise.

What would happen if you could eliminate the weak link in each of your lifts? Obviously, the amount of weight you could lift would increase dramatically because you would be able to move an increased amount of weight through the strong areas of the lifts.

The way to accomplish this is with power rack partials training. I will outline some workouts using this technique following an explanation of how and where to place the pins and when to add isometric training to the mix.

Using the bench press as an example, when you begin pressing the bar you will be able to move the weight well until you hit the middle zone, where the bar normally will stop moving. This is because your triceps, which are weaker than your chest become more involved in the lift and succumb to the weight much more quickly than your stronger pectoral muscles do.

To overcome this, we will place the pins in the rack at the point just before the sticking point begins and at the top portion of the sticking point. This allows us to focus our energies just on the sticking point section of the lift.

After loading the bar with a heavy weight, press the bar off the bottom pins until it hits the top pins. Continue to perform partial reps in this zone until you have exhausted your muscles and hit failure. Reduce the weight on the bar and repeat this sequence. After resting 30 seconds, repeat this sequence one last time. This is an example of the type of training we will be engaging in to improve our muscle strength and size.

Squat(Legs) Workout

Lockout squats- This improves your squat lockout. Set the bottom pins 6" before your legs are locked out in a squat. Load the bar with a heavier weight than you typically use in the squat. Do one set of 3 to failure. Rest one minute after reducing the weight and do a set of 5 reps to failure. Rest another minute then reduce the weight and do 8 reps to failure.

Bottom zone squats- Set the pins at the lowest point of the squat. Load the bar heavy and do one set of 3 to failure. Rest one minute after reducing the weight and do a set of 5 reps to failure. Rest another minute then reduce the weight and do 8 reps to failure.

Mid-range squats- Set the pins at the beginning of the middle zone and load the bar heavy. Do one set of 3 to failure. Rest one minute after reducing the weight and do a set of 5 reps to failure. Rest another minute then reduce the weight and do 8 reps to failure.

Isometric(Legs-Squat) Workout

Lockout isometric squat- Set the pins at the same point you placed them during the lockout exercise in the first workout. Load the bar near your 1RM. Squat the bar up and when it hits the top pin push as hard as you can for 20 seconds before resting the bar back on the lower pins. Rest for 20 seconds then repeat. Continue doing this sequence for a total of 8 single isometric reps. Note: It will be necessary to reduce the weight on every set.

Bottom zone isometric squat- Set the pins where you did during the bottom zone training in the first session. Load the bar with your 1RM or near that weight. Begin at the bottom and press hard against the top pins after contacting them for 20 seconds. Rest 20 seconds then repeat. Continue doing this sequence for a total of 8 single isometric reps. Note: It will be necessary to reduce the weight on every set.

Mid-range isometric squat- Set the pins at the middle zone. Load the bar with your 1RM or near that weight. Begin at the bottom pins and press hard against the top pins after contacting them for 20 seconds. Rest 20 seconds then repeat. Continue doing this sequence for a total of 8 single isometric reps. Note: It will be necessary to reduce the weight on every set.

Bench Press(Chest) Workout
Lockout bench press- Set the pins 6" from the lockout position and at the top. Load the bar with your 1RM and do one set of 3 to failure. Rest one minute after reducing the weight and do a set of 5 reps to failure. Rest another minute then reduce the weight and do 8 reps to failure.
Mid-range bench press- Set the pins at the beginning of the middle zone of the bench press and 6" above that. Load the bar with your 1RM and do one set of 3 to failure. Rest one minute after reducing the weight and do a set of 5 reps to failure. Rest another minute then reduce the weight and do 8 reps to failure.
Bottom zone bench press- Set the pins just above the beginning of the bench press and 6" above that. Load the bar with your 1RM and do one set of 3 to failure. Rest one minute after reducing the weight and do a set of 5 reps to failure. Rest another minute then reduce the weight and do 8 reps to failure.

Isometric(Chest-Bench press) Workout
Lockout isometric squat- Set the pins at the same point you placed them during the lockout exercise in the first workout. Load the bar near your 1RM. Press the bar up and when it hits the top pin push as hard as you can for 20 seconds before resting the bar back on the lower pins. Rest for 20 seconds then repeat. Continue doing this sequence for a total of 8 single isometric reps. Note: It will be necessary to reduce the weight on every set.
Mid-range isometric bench press- Set the pins at the beginning of the middle zone of the bench press and 6" above that. Load the bar with your 1RM or near that weight. Begin at the bottom pins and press hard against the top pins after contacting them for 20 seconds. Rest 20 seconds then repeat. Continue doing this sequence for a total of 8 single isometric reps. Note: It will be necessary to reduce the weight on every set.
Bottom zone isometric bench press- Set the pins just above the beginning of the bench press and 6" above that. Load the bar with your 1RM or near that weight. Begin at the bottom and press hard against the top pins after contacting them for 20 seconds. Rest 20 seconds then repeat. Continue doing this sequence for a total of 8 single isometric reps. Note: It will be necessary to reduce the weight on every set.

Deadlift(Back) Workout
Final zone deadlifts- Set the pins to restrict the movement of the bar to the final 6" of the deadlift. Load the bar to 90% of your 1RM. Assume a standard deadlift position with arms bent and legs wider than shoulder width. Use an over-underhand grip and lift the bar for 5 reps. Rest 30

seconds and do 8 reps after decreasing the weight. Rest another 30 seconds and do 5 reps after adjusting the weight. Rest 30 seconds and do 3 reps. **Middle zone deadlifts-** Set the pins to restrict the movement of the bar to the middle 12" of the deadlift. Load the bar to 90% of your 1RM. Assume a standard deadlift position with arms bent and legs wider than shoulder width. Use an over-underhand grip and lift the bar for 5 reps. Rest 30 seconds and do 8 reps after decreasing the weight. Rest another 30 seconds and do 5 reps after adjusting the weight. Rest 30 seconds and do 3 reps. **Beginning zone deadlifts-** Set the pins to restrict the movement of the bar to the beginning 12" of the deadlift. Load the bar to 90% of your 1RM. Assume a standard deadlift position with arms bent and legs wider than shoulder width. Use an over-underhand grip and lift the bar for 5 reps. Rest 30 seconds and do 8 reps after decreasing the weight. Rest another 30 seconds and do 5 reps after adjusting the weight. Finally rest 30 seconds and do 3 reps.

Isometric(Back-Deadlift) Workout

Final zone isometric deadlifts- Set the pins to restrict the movement of the bar to the final 6" of the deadlift. Load the bar with your 1RM or near that weight. Begin at the bottom and lift hard against the top pins after contacting them for 20 seconds. Rest 20 seconds then repeat. Continue doing this sequence for a total of 8 single isometric reps. Note: It will be necessary to reduce the weight on every set.

Middle zone isometric deadlifts- Set the pins at the beginning of the middle zone of the deadlift and 12" above that. Load the bar with your 1RM or near that weight. Begin at the bottom pins and lift hard against the top pins after contacting them for 20 seconds. Rest 20 seconds then repeat. Continue doing this sequence for a total of 8 single isometric reps. Note: It will be necessary to reduce the weight on every set.

Beginning zone isometric deadlifts- Set the pins to restrict the movement of the bar to the beginning 12" of the deadlift. Load the bar with your 1RM or near that weight. Begin at the bottom pins and lift hard against the top pins after contacting them for 20 seconds. Rest 20 seconds then repeat. Continue doing this sequence for a total of 8 single isometric reps. Note: It will be necessary to reduce the weight on every set.

These workouts should be combined. In other words, do the deadlift standard session first then the isometric one. Do the same for the two other lifts. You can also combine the two into one session, doing several partial reps and finishing your workout off with isometric reps.

If you have sticking points in other portions, or zones of a lift, feel free to modify the range of motion that you use in the lift. Instead of using the beginning 12" range in the deadlift you can change it to the 8"-15" range and work through the sticking point in that area. The same goes for all of the lifts.

Power rack partials and isometrics- assistance exercises

There are many great exercises available to train with using a power rack. These exercises are great for training the muscles that assist in performing the powerlifts, squat, deadlift and bench press.

The trap muscles of the shoulder- upper back region is an important muscle group for the deadlift. To train these muscles using a power rack we will use the upright rows and shrug lifts. A sample workout using these exercises is as follows:

Barbell shrugs- beginning zone- Set the pins so the bar only travels 6" from the start. Load the bar very heavy as it is possible to use very heavy weight in this exercise. Do a set of 6 partials, rest 30 seconds then continue with a set of 4 reps and a final set of two reps.
Barbell shrugs- end zone- Set the pins to limit movement to the last 4" in the final zone. Load the bar very heavy and do a set of 8 partials, rest 30 seconds and continue with a set of 6 partials. Reduce the weight on the bar and do a set of 4 partials. Reduce the weight again and complete a set of 2 partials.
Barbell shrugs- middle zone- Train this zone using the format as the end zone after you set the pins to limit movement to 8" in the middle of the exercise.

This format can be done with barbell rows for the back, or deadlift, incline or decline bench press for the chest, or bench press and leg presses for the legs, or squat. The power rack is one of the most versatile tools in the gym. Not only can it make lifting safer by "spotting" you during a lift, but it can help you overcome sticking points and improve your strength.

Additional Methods to Overcome Stagnation in Your Training

After you have been training for a while, you will hit a plateau and gains in fitness, strength and muscle size will stall. This is because your body is adept at conserving energy and adapting to stresses placed upon it. It costs a lot of energy, calories and nutrients to build new muscle tissue let alone maintain it and your body would rather maintain the status quo and not add tissue to your muscles. Luckily, there are several tools available to help you avoid these extended ruts and continue to make gains. One of these tools is Chaos Training. Blitz training is a related method of shocking muscles back to growth and will be explained here as well.

The following methods have been proven to be very effective. Use them to your advantage.

Chaos Training

This method works by structuring a workout that confuses the muscles, causing them to grow. Ways to do that include altering the rep cadence from one set to the next, changing the rep count (tut) on each set and switching the exercise sequence.

Three different workouts (for any exercise) using a rest-pause style of exercise as well as other techniques are as follows:

WORKOUT 1
3 repetitions (5/5 cadence)
10-second rest
3 repetitions (5/5 cadence)
5-second rest
1 repetition at a slow 10/5
cadence followed by...
8 top partials + 1 forced rep

WORKOUT 2
3 repetitions (5/5 cadence)
10-second rest
4 repetitions (3/4 cadence)
0 second rest
4 negatives, followed by 10
second static hold at bottom

WORKOUT 3
3 repetitions (5/5 cadence)
15-second rest
8 repetitions (3/3 cadence)
0 second rest
2 forced, followed by 1 set of pec
deck x 5 reps

The chaos method can also be applied to traditional sets where a trainee completes a typical rep count before integrating set variables that modify the rest of the set. For example, before performing forced reps, negative reps, partials, static holds, etc., a trainee would complete six repetitions at a particular cadence and TUT, for instance, 2 second positive, 4 second negative- 2/4 with a time under tension of 36 seconds.

At each workout the trainee would increase the weight by 5 pounds while maintaining the same cadence and rep scheme but he/she would integrate HIT variables into the set. This gives the trainee a new and interesting way in which to stimulate the muscles and to maintain motivation.

Chaos prioritizing

In the table below the shoulders receive priority in Workout 1 with the military press, the chest receives priority in Workout 2 and the back receives priority in Workout 3.

This sequence is repeated for five cycles before moving on to the next block of five cycles, which focuses on a different scheme of prioritization. The only workouts being compared to each other are those that include the same beginning exercise.

The back workout, for example, will be based only on Workout 3 in Cycles 1-5. Although improvement is possible in the other workouts, it is difficult to speculate as to what extent, or how well the trainee has performed, since the non-back exercises performed previously influence the outcome of the back exercises performed after.

Cycles 1-5 (workouts 1-3 = one cycle)
Workout 1: Deltoid Emphasis
Military Press
Nautilus Flyes + Pushups
Seated Row
Nautilus Torso

Workout 2: Pectoral Emphasis
Chest Press
Dip
Pulldown
Deadlift/Shrug

Workout 3: Back Emphasis
Nautilus Pulldown
Dumbbell Press
Bar Dips
Lateral Raise
Cycles 6-10 (workouts 4-6 = one cycle)

Workout 4: Pectoral Emphasis
Nautilus Flyes + Pushups
Nautilus Torso
Seated Row
Military Press

Workout 5: Back Emphasis
Deadlift/Shrug
Pulldown
Dip
Chest Press

Workout 6: Deltoid Emphasis
Lateral Raise
Dips
Dumbbell Press
Pulldown

Blitz

A blitz program is designed to "shock" the muscles into new growth. When the body becomes accustomed to a training routine that has been performed steadily with no or very little changes it stops growing or adding muscle mass. By radically changing the workout and increasing either set volume, intensity or both for a short period of time, growth can start again. The following program is an example of this:

WEEK 1 BLITZ

SUNDAY
Thighs: Tri-set 12-15 reps each + 4 forced reps (no rest between exercises) – leg extensions, squat, sissy squat
two minute rest
leg curls- 2 sets of 15 reps (+ burns).
Repeat two times.

TUESDAY
Deltoids: Side lateral raises with dumbbells 8-10 reps
one-minute rest
bent-over lateral raises (quadruple breakdown with 5 seconds rest between mini-sets)- do a set of 8 reps to failure then reduce the weight 25%- do more reps to failure. Repeat for a total of four mini-sets.

One-minute rest

Front dumbbell raises (quadruple breakdown with 15 seconds between mini-sets).
The quadruple breakdowns are done as follows: do reps to failure, set the dumbbells down and grab the next lightest pair and rep to failure. That constitutes 2 mini-sets. Do two more mini-sets for a total of four.

Abs: Machine crunch (triple drop set)
Dumbbell side bends (single set each side)

Upper Arms: Machine curls and Dips- two sets 8-10 reps each of forced overloads.

To do an overload, have a partner add enough resistance to the movement arm during both the positive and negative portions to make them maximum efforts. As the set progresses, he/she will need to reduce the amount of pressure due to your muscular fatigue.
Forearms/Grip: Grip hold (pinch grip a heavy barbell plate and hold it several inches above the floor for as long as you can)
Wrist curl (sets of 12 reps + burns partial reps at the end of the set)
Reverse wrist curl (sets of 12 reps + burns partial reps at the end of the set)
Do a total of 3 supersets.

THURSDAY
Back: High row (double breakdown with 15 seconds rest between mini-sets)
two minutes rest
Machine row (quadruple breakdown)
two minutes rest
Hyperextension (single set + one 20-second static hold)
two minutes rest
Pulldown 3 sets (one set each of overhand, neutral, and underhand position).

SATURDAY
Chest: Machine press (triple drop with 20 seconds rest between mini-sets)
two minutes rest
Parallel bar dips (one rest pause set consisting of 8 reps + 5 negatives at the end of the final set)
supersetted with Nautilus ten-degree flyes (triple drop)
two minutes rest
Bodyweight pushups (straight set + 5 negatives).

WEEK 2 BLITZ

MONDAY
Thighs: Tri-set (minimal rest) leg extension-one set of 15 reps
Front squat-12 reps
Sissy squat-12 reps + 4 forced reps
Pendulum leg curl -triple drop set + burn reps

WEDNESDAY
Arms: Triceps pushdowns- 8 reps
Bench dips-10 reps
Preacher cable curls-10 reps
Close-grip pulldowns-8 reps
Do a total of three giant sets

Forearms/Grip: Reverse cable preacher curl-8 reps (triple
breakdown set with 5 seconds rest between minisets)
One-minute rest
Preacher cable wrist curl- one set of 15 reps
Do a total of three supersets

FRIDAY
Deltoids: Lateral raise-one set of 10 reps
Dumbbell press-one set of 10 reps
One-minute rest
Bent over lateral raise-one set of 10 reps
Dumbbell press-one set of 8 reps
Rotator cuff rotations-12 reps
Do two giant sets with 90 seconds rest in between them

Abs: Machine crunch (triple drop with 15 seconds
between mini-sets).

SUNDAY
Chest: Machine bench press- 1 set of 8 forced negative reps
Dips-1 set 8 reps negative-only
Pushups-1 set to failure
Rest one minute then repeat for a total of two supersets

Back: Seated row (up and down method)
Single arm pulldowns- 1 set of 10 reps plus 4 forced reps per side
Deadlift-1 set of 8 reps performed rest pause style

Many different combinations can be used with this program. The important point to remember is to limit this program to 2-3 weeks.

HIIT Training – The Superior Way to Cardiovascular Health

When you typically think of aerobic training you naturally think of jogging, swimming and other similar exercises.

But recently a newer form of aerobic training has been gaining in popularity.

HIIT, or high intensity interval training, differs from low-moderate intensity aerobic training such as jogging in that it condenses all of the effort into short bursts of maximum effort with brief rest periods in between.

Typically people who jog do so for 5 miles or more 3-5 times per week using a low to moderate pace. This is considered low intensity aerobic training. If enough effort is put forth, this training can result in substantial fat loss if an appropriate diet is undertaken.

But research has shown that the same amount or more calories are burned during a HIIT, High Intensity Interval Training session even though a session lasts, in many cases, only 15-20 minutes, two-three times per week.

To try a HIIT version of aerobic training perform the following routine using running (sprinting) as an example:

- Warm up with brisk walking for 2 minutes followed by a moderate jog for one minute.
- Sprint with as near 100% effort as you can for 20 seconds
- Walk briskly for 1 ½ minutes
- Sprint for 20 seconds
- Walk briskly for 1 ½ minutes

Repeat this for one more cycle. After the last cycle do a cool down period of moderate walking for two minutes.

Do this training twice per week during the initial month. It's a good idea to have three rest days between workouts to allow your muscles and central nervous system time to fully recuperate. If you find that you are dragging when you attempt to repeat the training, add a rest day before resuming. This will allow you to build up your tolerance for this type of training over a safe timeframe. During the second month increase your sessions by doing a total of 5 cycles per session. Repeat this routine three times per week.

A very effective method for increasing the effectiveness of this type of training is to vary both the rest periods and the short bursts of effort. For instance, try doing a 15 second sprint with a one-minute rest period in between or a 10 second sprint with a 45 second rest period. This is a great way to keep your exercise interesting and avoid boredom. Set goals for yourself and remember you get results based on the effort put forth!

A kickboxing routine using HIIT

Kickboxing training is an excellent way to use HIIT Training to improve your cardio conditioning and have fun doing it! Because you are punching and kicking against a heavy bag and other reflex bags, you are getting some resistance effect which helps in building muscle while at the same time you are getting great cardio stimulation from all of the equipment you are using.

This training is a great alternative to boring, time-intensive cardio such as endless jogging on a treadmill or streets and low-intensive training on elliptical machines. Treadmills and elliptical machines are great tools, but the way they are used in most gyms, incorrectly, lessens the benefits that can be derived from them. Most of the time you will see people watching TV on the built-in screens while they keep themselves at a slower pace.

I am going to outline an effective cardio-conditioning program for you that merges the equipment used in kickboxing with a stationary bicycle, elliptical and treadmill.

Definition of Terms

Roundhouse kick- Stand facing the heavy bag sideways. Spin toward the bag and kick it with the instep of your foot.
Side kick- Stand sideways to the heavy bag. Lift your leg and kick the bag out to your side.
Front kick- Face the heavy bag, lift your leg straight up and kick the bag.

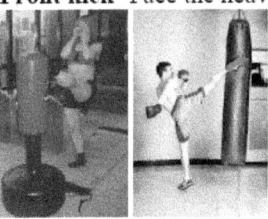
front kick   roundhouse kick

Round- Time of training. Generally we train in each phase using a three-minute round.

When training during the round go with 100% effort, holding nothing back. You will have to work up to this level of effort especially if you haven't achieved a high level of conditioning to this point.

Workout#1
3-minute round- Punch and kick the heavy bag using straight and circular punches, roundhouse, front and side kicks.
Rest one minute
3-minute round- Stationary bicycle
Rest one minute
3-minute round- Punch and kick the heavy bag using straight and circular punches, roundhouse, front and side kicks.
Rest one minute
3-minute round-Treadmill- Begin by running on a flat level and increasing the elevation. Don't adjust the height too much; the main thing we are looking for is the percentage of effort you are able to exert.
Rest one minute
3-minute round- Elliptical machine
Rest one minute
3-minute round- Punch and kick the punching ball using straight and circular punches, roundhouse, front and side kicks.

Keep in mind this is an advanced workout-one that must be worked up to. If you begin too quickly you will injure yourself or become too sore the next few days after training. Not that some sore muscles is a bad thing-just don't overdue it the first few times you train. An ideal way to break into this routine is to begin by doing the first few rounds of training and adding more as you progress over a 4-6 week time period.

Workout#2
3-minute round- Punch and kick the heavy bag using straight and circular punches, roundhouse, front and side kicks.
Rest one minute
3-minute round- Punch the speed bag using different punches like straight jabs and right and left crosses. Change the tempo of the punches but keep a steady fast speed through the round.
Rest one minute
3-minute round- Punch the speed ball, which should be located at sternum height. Use various combinations of punches and vary the combinations of punches. For instance, do a couple of single punches with each hand then a quick three punch combination using both hands. Get creative and have fun.

Rest one minute

3-minute round- Punch the reflex ball using different combinations of punches like you did with the speed ball during the last round.

Rest one minute

3-minute round- Punch and kick the heavy bag using straight and circular punches, roundhouse, front and side kicks.

After each workout routine do several minutes of cool down by performing slow punches and kicks on the heavy bag. The idea is to wind down your HIIT training by bringing your energy level back to normal after the vigorous activity.

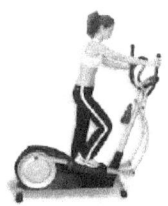 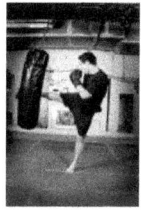

Isolation and Compound weight training exercises

The following is a list of isolation (single joint) and compound (multi-joint) exercises for each muscle group:

Legs-compound- squat, leg press, dumbbell squat, sissy squat, hack squat, lunge
Isolation- leg extension, leg curl, calf raise, seated calf raise, donkey calf raise, toe presses on leg press machine
Back-compound- barbell/dumbbell rows, end barbell rows, machine rows, pulldowns, deadlift, stiff-legged deadlifts, good mornings, kettlebell swings, pull-up, chin-up
Isolation- Stiff-arm pulldown, dumbbell pullovers, machine pullovers, ab strap bent arm pulldowns, seated reverse machine flyes, Nautilus behind neck machine, side cable lat pulldowns
Chest- compound- bench press, incline bench press, decline bench press, dumbbell bench press, incline dumbbell bench press, decline dumbbell bench press, push-ups
Isolation- dumbbell flyes, incline dumbbell flyes, decline dumbbell flyes, low pulley cable crossovers, mid pulley cable crossovers, high pulley cable crossovers, band low flyes, band mid flyes, band high flyes, pek dek, machine flyes
Shoulders- compound- barbell presses, dumbbell presses, band presses, snatch, clean and jerk

Isolation- Front deltoid raise, side deltoid raise, bent-over deltoid raise, front cable raise, side cable raise, bent-over cable raise, dumbbell rotations, upright rows, seated machine lateral raise, Arnold press, band pull-apart, cable internal rotation, face pull

Biceps- compound- cable pulldowns, bent-over forward grip rows, palms-up cable row

Isolation- barbell curl, dumbbell curl, cable curl, band curl, preacher curl, concentration curl, incline dumbbell curl, bench dumbbell curl, single-arm rope curl behind neck, two-arm rope curls behind neck, rope curl, lying bar curl, lying rope curl, hammer curl, machine curl, barbell reverse curl, reverse machine curl, zottman curl, cross-body hammer curl, drag curl

Triceps- compound- close-grip bench press, bar dips, bench dips, machine dips, narrow push-ups

Isolation- cable pressdown, reverse-grip cable pressdown, cable pushdown, rope pressdown, seated dumbell tricep extension, lying tricep extension, machine tricep extension, standing 30-degree cable tricep extension, dumbbell tricep kickback

Forearms- isolation- barbell wrist curl, dumbbell wrist curl, barbell reverse wrist curl, rope wind-ups, grip squeeze, reverse grip squeeze, ball squeeze, side forearm rotation, side reverse forearm rotation, plate pinch grip, barbell finger curl, one-sided dumbell wrist rotations

Abdominals- isolation- sit-ups, ab crunches, ab machine crunches, ab wheel roll, lying leg raises, hanging leg raises, machine leg raises, inversion bench sit-ups, side rotations, side machine rotations

Bonus section

Answers to your questions

Can I reduce fat on my midsection quickly with a lot of sit-ups or crunches?
While doing sit-ups and crunches burns calories, there is no such thing as spot reduction. The best method to lose weight around your core, or midsection, is to eat a clean diet and train the large muscles of your body such as legs, back and chest. This is because these muscles are the biggest in the body therefore they burn the most energy, or calories, during exercise. Do your ab training to tighten and strengthen the muscles in that area but do compound exercises like squats, leg presses, bench presses, etc to burn large amounts of calories. Remember larger muscles burn more calories so by building muscle you increase your calorie burn. One of the best methods to burn fat is cardio, preferably the HIIT variety. This burns fat in a short amount of time, reducing the chances of boredom creeping in.

I see most people really swing the kettlebell while doing kettlebell swings. Sometimes they can barely handle the weight but use momentum to swing heavy weights. Is this dangerous?
Yes. While the name kettlebell swings seems to suggest a recommendation to forcefully swing the kettlebell weight up this is dangerous and counterproductive for a couple of reasons. When momentum is used to swing a weight up the muscle isn't subjected to nearly as much workload as when the weight is controlled by the muscle.

A study showed that by using momentum to move a weight you are subjecting your muscles, bones and tendons to very dangerous amounts of stress. In fact, it was proven that the amount of stress on your body is ten times what it normally is while training properly. So be careful and do a kettlebell swing with an appropriate weight under your own power, with no momentum.

Are weight machines able to build muscle or do I need to use free weights instead? Great question. Many bodybuilders and powerlifters feel that the only way to build muscle mass is to use free weights only. Weight machines are believed to be only good for shaping a muscle.

The truth is that resistance in any form lends itself toward building muscle tissue if the exercise is performed correctly at the proper intensity level using proper techniques. The main difference between free weights is not which one builds the most muscle tissue but in how they are used to advantage.

The advantage in using free weights is the building of functional strength and balance, especially if dumbbells are used. They certainly have their drawbacks but they mimic the body's own movements the closest. The downside to free weights is the exercises feature angles that don't maximize the resistance to the muscles.

A great example of this is the barbell or dumbbell curl. When you begin the curl, the resistance on your biceps is strong and continues to increase until peaking at the mid-point. It then fades until all of the weight is removed from your biceps at the top, making the point where contraction should be highest worthless for building muscle.

Properly designed weight machines compensate for this imperfection in the curl by way of a specially designed cam that varies the resistance throughout the movement to correspond with the strength curves of each individual muscle, whether it be a bicep, tricep, thigh, back or any other muscle of the body. Machines also force you to move the machine's arms in the proper groove to follow the natural path of the muscle being trained.

So my answer to the question is to use both forms of equipment thereby maximizing the results you receive from your training efforts. Use free weights for both compound and isolation exercises to grow and tone muscle and use machines for the same purpose. Preference will dictate which you will use more of, but learn the proper methods to use both.

What are advantages, if any, to using bands for training?
Bands have become very popular for fitness use and continue to increase in popularity as time goes on. The reason for this is their effectiveness as a stand-alone piece of equipment for fitness training and strength building.

They add a unique feel to your training and have been used extensively by power lifters as a way to build explosiveness to their lifts. This is done by hooking the one end of the band to an attachment on the base of a power rack and attaching the other end to a special collar on a barbell. In the bench press, for example, as the bar is pressed higher the band stretches and increases the resistance on the bar. This demands the lifter press harder as the lift progresses, which is invaluable in a power lifting competition.

How can you use them in your training? Well, you can use them in a similar fashion as power lifters do but you can also use them by themselves in your training.

Using squats as an example, step on one end of the band with both feet and loop the other end over both shoulders. Squat down as far as you can and drive yourself up against the resistance of the band. This can also be performed one leg at a time. Use a lighter resistance band and do a one-legged band squat. This allows you to isolate the leg being worked so more attention can be focused on it.

There are many unique exercises that can be done with bands. Refer to the section in this book for a number of great exercise routines using this great tool!

Is it possible to gain muscle and strength after 40?
Yes! While the gains won't come as fast or to the degree that they do at a younger age, it is possible to gain both muscle size and strength even at ages much more advanced than 40.

This attests to the possibilities that weight training adds to your life, whether it be with free weights, bands, machines or some other tool. Just remember to begin slowly as old injuries can be aggravated by new exercise and be sure to clear your new training program with your physician.

If you are just beginning training begin slowly to break-in your muscles otherwise you will experience extreme soreness in the muscles you trained. Train using good form in all exercises as I have stressed in this book and you should successfully avoid injuries.

Begin with a good basic program using both compound and isolation exercises for each muscle group. Do 1-2 total sets per body part ending each set one or two reps before muscle exhaustion. Once you have become used to working out and are using proper form on all your exercises increase the intensity by ending all sets at muscular exhaustion, or failure. Train your large muscles first and work down to the smaller muscles like arms at the end of your workout as they already receive a lot of stimulation from compound exercises used to train the larger muscles such as chest and back. Use the workout programs in this and my other books and you will make great progress.

My contact information: http://www.personal-resistance-trainer.com
daverg@verizon.net

My High Intensity Training Blog: http://drhitshighintensitybodybuilding.blogspot.com/

www.ingramcontent.com/pod-product-compliance
Lightning Source LLC
Chambersburg PA
CBHW070926290526
45795CB00001B/445